Resources for Elders

with

Disabilities

Resources for Rehabilitation
Winchester, Massachusetts

Resources for Rehabilitation
22 Bonad Road
Winchester, MA 01890
(781) 368-9094   FAX (781) 368-9096
e-mail: info@rfr.org www.rfr.org

Resources for Elders with Disabilities, fifth edition
ISBN 0-929718-31-3

Copyright 2003 by Resources for Rehabilitation, Inc.

Library of Congress Cataloging-in-Publication Data

Resources for elders with disabilities.-- 5th ed.
    p. cm.
Includes bibliographical references and index.
  ISBN 0-929718-31-3 (pbk. : alk. paper)
 1. Aged people with disabilities--Care--United States. 2. Aged people with disabilities--Rehabilitation--United States. 3. Aged people with disabilities--Medical care--United States. I. Resources for Rehabilitation (Organization)
  RA564.8 .R47 2002
  362.4'048'0846--dc21

                              2002012971

For a description of other publications from Resources for Rehabilitation, see pages 332-336 362.4048
R4336

TABLE OF CONTENTS

HOW TO USE THIS BOOK

This book was written to inform elders, family members, caregivers, and professional service providers about the many organizations, services, and assistive devices that contribute to the independence of elders with disabilities. Although these services and products have expanded greatly in recent years, many elders and service providers alike are confused by the vast array of services and their eligibility criteria. Still others are unaware of the many opportunities available to help elders maintain their independence.

Because individuals have different lifestyles, needs, and degrees of impairment, this book is organized so that readers may select the services and devices that are most appropriate to their specific needs. Each chapter includes an introductory narrative, information about organizations that provide services to elders with disabilities, and information about relevant publications and tapes. Chapters that deal with specific health conditions (e.g., arthritis, diabetes, hearing loss, etc.) describe causes and effects of the condition or impairment and common psychological responses as well as include information about professional service providers; where to find services; and assistive devices.

Descriptions of organizations, publications and tapes, and assistive devices are alphabetical within sections. Most publications are available at bookstores and libraries. For those readers who would like to purchase the publications listed, the address and phone number of the publisher or distributor are included. Only directories that have timely information and those that are updated regularly are included. All of the material is up-to-date, and prices were accurate at the time of publication. However, it is always advisable to contact publishers and manu-facturers to inquire about availability and current prices as well as shipping and handling charges.

Developments in computer technology, such as the Internet and e-mail, have greatly increased access to information for the general population as well as people with disabilities and chronic conditions. Internet addresses are provided for organizations when available.

The use of "TTY" in the listings indicates a teletypewriter, a special telephone system for individuals who are deaf or have hearing impairments and those who have speech impairments (also known as a "TDD," telecommunication device for the deaf or "TT," text telephone). The use of "V/TTY" indicates that the same telephone number is used for both voice and TTY. Toll-free numbers may begin with "800," "888," "877," or "866."

The phrase "alternate formats" in the listings indicates that, in addition to standard print, publications may also be available in large print, audiocassette, braille, or disk.

Chapter 1

OUR AGING SOCIETY

Improvement in medical technology and living conditions has resulted in increased longevity in modern society. In the United States, 35 million elders, defined as those age 65 or above, now comprise 12.4% of the population (Administration on Aging: 2001). It is projected that this population will increase rapidly in the future; the population of 34.1 million Americans age 65 or older in 1997 is projected to grow to 69.4 million in the year 2030, or 20% of the population (American Association of Retired Persons: 1998).

The older an individual is, the more likely it is that he or she will have a disability. Among Americans age 65 or older, 54.5% had a disability, with 37.7% having a severe disability. For those ages 65 to 69, 44.9% had a disability, and 30.7% had a severe disability in 1997. For those Americans age 80 or older, 73.6% had a disability, and 57.6%0 had a severe disability in 1997 (McNeil: 2001). Since the 85 and over group is the most rapidly growing sub-group within the older population (American Association of Retired Persons: 1998), it is apparent that the number of elders with disabilities will continue to increase. The increase in the older population will create a need for increased services and assistance that enable elders to carry out the tasks of everyday living.

To accommodate the rapid increase in the number of elders, there has been a proliferation of services and products in both the private and public sectors. Federal legislation has engendered a hierarchy of aging agencies at the regional, state, and local levels. While many agencies focus on healthy elders, others provide services for elders who have one or more disabilities.

For example, many hospitals have established special departments for older adults. Home care and long term care organizations offer a variety of service options to elders. Private consultants, often working as case coordinators, offer services to individuals and families. Many public libraries have special programs for elders, people with disabilities, and people who are homebound. And agencies that had traditionally focused on younger clients, such as vocational rehabilitation agencies, have had to re-evaluate their services in light of the growing number of elders with disabilities.

In 1997, over 4.5 million elders reported having difficulties in carrying out activities of everyday living, which include bathing, dressing, and eating, and 6.9 million reported difficulties with instrumental activities of everyday living, defined as getting around outside the home, keeping track of money and bills, preparing meals, doing light housework, and using the telephone (McNeil: 2001).

Most elders have at least one chronic condition, and many elders have multiple conditions. Despite the high rate of chronic conditions, most elders live in the community, with nearly a third living alone, and only 5% live in nursing homes (U.S. Department of Health and Human Services: 1991).

ELDERS AND DISABILITIES

A disability changes a person's life dramatically. To many members of society, people with physical impairments bear a stigma; their social status has decreased, and they become the objects of others' curiosity. People with disabilities are aware of the way in which society views them. As a result, some people try to "pass" or to hide their disabilities. Many individuals who experience their first physical impairment in later life once held the same stereotypes that they now fear will be applied to them. Because our society has traditionally been "ageist" as well, elders with disabilities bear a double stigma.

Elders also hold misconceptions about what it means to be old. Too many elders associate pain, discomfort, debilitation, or decline in intellectual function with aging per se. The notion that disabilities are to be expected as a function of aging deters many

10

individuals from seeking out services. Elders' functional abilities may be more accurate indicators of their potential than the presence or absence of illness or impairments. For instance, some people with poor visual acuity function better than those whose measured visual acuity is better.

It has been suggested that elders who attribute physical symptoms to the natural course of aging are unlikely to take measures to remediate these symptoms. At the same time, research has shown that interventions may increase elders' sense of control, lessening their sense that decline is inevitable with aging and therefore unremediable (Rodin: 1989).

The roles of professional service providers may be crucial in shaping elders' responses to disability, yet several studies have shown that service providers often fail to tell elders about organizations and products that can help them cope with their disabilities. For example, Greenblatt's (1991) study of individuals who had experienced vision loss found that many had not received the information they needed to obtain rehabilitation services. An earlier study had indicated that a large proportion of ophthalmologists are not aware of many of the services that can help their patients with vision loss (Greenblatt: 1988). Research in other fields has also found that service providers neglect to refer elders for services; for example, otologists, otolaryngologists, and family physicians often do not refer older patients with hearing losses for aural rehabilitation (Glass and Elliott: 1992; Taylor: 1991).

Professionals can help people with disabilities to continue functioning in socially productive roles and to avoid the feeling that they need to "pass." Combating professionals' negative attitudes toward elders with disabilities is an essential first step in serving this growing population.

PSYCHOLOGICAL RESPONSES TO DISABILITY

It is commonly accepted that disability results in depression. Less attention has been paid to the possibility that depression may result in disability. A study of elders living in the community (age 70 to 79) found that depression and disability combined to create a downward spiral of the ability to carry out activities of daily living. Over the two and a half year period in which the study was carried out, those elders who started out with no disabilities were more likely to have an onset of disability if they were depressed (Bruce: 1994).

It is normal for people who have experienced a disability to go through a series of emotions including depression, denial, bargaining, anger, and acceptance. These reactions are similar to those that occur after other losses, such as the death of a loved one. Not every individual experiences all of these reactions. Some people may be chronically depressed; some may deny the permanency or severity of their loss; others may accept the loss and move on to acceptance of rehabilitation services and assistive aids or devices.

An individual's reactions may be shaped by the severity of the loss and whether it occurs suddenly or gradually. Knowledge of the person's previous reactions to stressful situations may provide insight into his or her responses to disabling conditions. It is common to rely on coping mechanisms that have been developed over a course of a lifetime. Religious faith, family, and friends may help elders to face disability and cope with it in a positive manner.

With the sudden onset of disability, the individual may be in a state of shock. Depression, the most common response to loss, often follows shock. Both shock and depression are normal precedents to emotional recovery. Depression is not always recognized, because it may be masked by weakness, apathy, irritability, and passivity (Hollander: 1982). Denial of the presence of the disability is also a common reaction. Individuals with chronic impairments must not be encouraged to believe that their condition will be reversed. They must fully accept their loss before emotional recovery can occur. Individuals who deny their disabilities should be referred for counseling, as it is unlikely that rehabilitation will be effective at this stage.

When the onset of disability is gradual and early intervention measures are taken, the individual may be motivated to learn new ways of accomplishing ordinary tasks. In addition, the individual may be better able to handle depression; may retain a positive self-image; and strive to be independent.

Some disabling conditions, such as arthritis and osteoporosis, cause pain as well as disability. Elders' attitudes toward pain may affect their willingness to accept rehabilitation or medication. Chronic pain may prevent elders from participating in rehabilitation activities. A desire to "tough it out" or a fear of addiction may influence their responses to questions about their pain levels. Cultural attitudes toward pain, especially among elders, are often unrecognized by health care personnel. While some cultures believe that expressing feelings of pain is taboo, others sanction free expression of pain. These beliefs may lead health care professionals to overestimate or underestimate an individual's pain tolerance and affect the prescription of pain control medications.

On the other hand, a common feature of ageism among physicians is prescribing too many medications. Elders who take a variety of medications may find that the interaction of the various drugs causes unpleasant side effects, and some may cause what appears to be mental confusion or impairment. Physicians frequently prescribe psychotropic drugs (antianxiety drugs, anti-depressants, or sedatives) to older patients, believing that they will quell patients' anxieties. Often, however, these drugs deprive elders of their mental alertness, which in turn may increase depression.

In 1998, the American Geriatrics Society released clinical practice guidelines for the management of chronic pain in elders.

The guidelines include recommendations on the assessment of chronic pain, pharmacologic treatments, and nonpharmacologic strategies, and the obligations of the health care system to provide comfort and pain management (American Geriatrics Society: 1998). Elders who experience chronic pain may wish to consider maintaining a pain diary in which they record pain episodes; intensity; use of medications and their effectiveness; nonpharmacologic interventions such as applying heat or cold, massage, or relaxation techniques; and activities associated with the pain episode. This pain history will help develop a course of treatment.

An elder's sensory losses may affect his or her ability to properly administer medications. If it is difficult to hear oral instructions and to read the tiny print on a pill bottle, the elder is at risk for misusing the medication. Memory loss may account for errors in under-or over-medication. Many of the drugs commonly taken by elders for heart conditions or high blood pressure may cause depression.

WHERE TO FIND LOCAL SERVICES

There is a wide variety of services available to elders in most areas. A good place to start the search for services is the information and referral office of the local United Way. State offices on aging or elder affairs and state offices established to serve people with disabilities are other sources of referrals. Many municipalities also have special offices to serve elders and individuals with disabilities. Other sources of information are local directories of service agencies available in the reference collection of many public libraries. Libraries often have special programs for elders, and some have special needs centers or special reading equipment for people with visual impairments.

Many hospitals have established special programs for elders, as have visiting nurse associations and home care agencies. Senior centers often provide special services for elders with disabilities. Churches and synagogues sometimes administer special programs for elders. Medical schools and universities that have special training programs for geriatricians and gerontologists may be able to make appropriate referrals. In many communities, special shopping services are available where individuals may phone in orders and have their groceries delivered to their homes.

Veterans are eligible for special benefits and rehabilitation services. In the United States, the Department of Veterans Affairs (VA) has established special services for aging veterans, including nursing home units and adult day care centers designed to provide rehabilitation and health care that prevent institutionalization. Prosthetics are provided for veterans with service related disabilities. Visual Impairment Services Teams (VIST) help veterans with vision loss at many VA Medical Centers across the country. The VA will specially adapt the homes of veterans with disabilities. Since the 1970's, the VA has established Geriatric Research, Education and Clinical Centers (GRECCs) at some VA Medical Centers across the country.

REHABILITATION

The rehabilitation process helps individuals who have irreversible impairments or chronic disabling conditions to continue functioning in society. Rehabilitation is appropriate when medical and surgical interventions are incapable of restoring the individual's functioning to normal. Rehabilitation includes counseling; training in new skills for daily activities; adapting the physical environment in which the individual works and lives; and the provision of special equipment that enables the individual to continue functioning. It may also include arrangements for social contacts through activities such as adult day health programs, recreation programs, volunteer opportunities, and senior citizen centers. Those elders who wish to continue working should receive vocational rehabilitation services as well.

Rehabilitation was originally intended for adults who were to be trained or retrained for employment situations and for youths who were in school. Some studies (cited in Benedict and Ganikos: 1981) have indicated that rehabilitation professionals exhibit evidence of ageism. Because the proportion of the population with disabilities has increasingly shifted to the older population in recent years, agencies that provide rehabilitation services have been mandated to re-evaluate the services they offer and to consider homemaking and independent living as appropriate goals of rehabilitation.

Independent living programs enable people with disabilities to continue functioning within the community with a minimal amount of assistance. For some, this means living at home (with or without homemaker assistance) and maintaining employment. For others, it means congregate living, where each person has his or her own apartment but eats in a communal dining room. And for others, it means shared living situations, where elders are matched with one another and share expenses and responsibilities in a private home. Individuals with severe disabilities often require assistance with personal care, transportation, and special equipment. Independent living programs or centers are sometimes administered by rehabilitation agencies, or they may be free-standing organizations administered by individuals with disabilities themselves.

Ideally, the approach to medical treatment and rehabilitation planning should be carried out jointly by health professionals and rehabilitation professionals. Because the medical profession is largely oriented toward cure rather than rehabilitation, such a collaborative approach is often a difficult goal to attain. The individual should have major input into the decision-making process regarding his or her rehabilitation. In fact, the federal government requires that individuals sign an Individual Written Rehabilitation Program that indicates they approve of the rehabilitation strategy developed jointly with counselors in state rehabilitation agencies.

It is important to involve family members in the rehabilitation process so that they will support, not undermine, the person's attempts to remain independent. It is not unusual for an elder to complete a rehabilitation program, only to return home to an over-protective family that interferes with the use of newly acquired skills. In some cases, it may be the elder with a disability who uses the situation to increase dependence upon a spouse or offspring. Family members who provide support to elders who are undergoing rehabilitation may make a valuable contribution to a positive rehabilitation outcome. In either situation, counseling with a social worker or psychologist may help to change family dynamics and result in greater independence.

SELF-HELP GROUPS

Self-help groups enable individuals with similar problems or conditions to discuss their problems and offer mutual assistance. Self-help groups offer a number of benefits to participants, including learning to develop coping strategies; acquiring a sense of control over their lives; combating isolation and alienation; and developing networks. In addition, members of self-help groups often express a sense of increased self-esteem, because they have offered help to other members of the group.

Self-help group members often believe that their peers are more understanding and patient than professional counselors, health care providers, or even family members, because they have had similar experiences. The person who needs help may feel weak or incompetent, no matter what his or her profession or background. Receiving help from a peer tends to minimize these feelings.

Professionals who work with elders are ideally suited to identify and bring together individuals with common problems, and they often are able to offer a site where meetings may be held. However, professionals must understand the new role that they play in helping to create a self-help group. Madara (no date) recommends that professionals assume the role of consultants, providing advice and counsel but not assuming any responsibility for leadership, decision-making, or group tasks. A professional who is the catalyst for the formation of a group must disengage from this initial role to allow the group to develop autonomously. Since professionals often tend to encourage dependent client relationships, they must guard against this type of relationship if a group is to offer true mutual support.

Identifying a group facilitator or coordinator is the first step in developing a self-help group for elders with disabilities. One method is to identify someone who has had group experience. Former patients or clients who have had experience in coping with disabilities are likely candidates for starting a group. Another method, especially useful in rural areas where no groups or services are available, is to identify an organized, articulate person who has experienced a disability and has some background in a club or other organization. Announcements made in publications read by elders, at educational meetings, and posters on hospital and agency bulletin boards are also good recruitment techniques. Once the group is established, it is up to the members to decide how frequently to meet; the types of discussions or programs they would like to have; and how to recruit members.

FAMILY MEMBERS AS CAREGIVERS

The impact of acting as a caregiver cannot be overemphasized. The impact on the caregivers themselves is both physical and psychological. Caregivers who locate appropriate services for elders may enable them to continue living in the community independently. Especially for those age 85 or over, who are at greatest risk for placement in long term care facilities, the support provided by caregivers may be the key factor in avoiding institutionalization (Manton and Soldo: 1992). One study found that with the receipt of assistance from others, elders were more likely to provide their own self-care (Norburn et al.: 1995).

Family members often find themselves in the role of caregiver for an older relative or spouse and are required to take on additional roles. Caregivers in our society are most frequently women, who often have additional responsibilities both at home and at work. Adding the role of caregiver to an already overburdened lifestyle may result in great stress. Often the caregiver must take time away from his or her employment outside the home in order to carry out the necessary tasks. These tasks include provision of transportation, arranging for medical appointments, shopping and other household tasks, and supervising medication. In some cases, individuals 65 or older are also providing care not only for their spouses but also for their elderly parents (usually mothers) who may be 85 or older. These older caregivers may also be experiencing the effects of chronic health problems themselves, making caregiving more difficult. In some cases, well meaning caregivers may try to do too much for their relatives, resulting in the relatives losing confidence in their ability to act independently. The natural concern that some offspring feel for parents with disabilities may, if carried too far, be detrimental. As a possible solution, Tinetti and Powell (1993) suggest that family members be included in assessment and treatment plans for their relatives.

Caregiving for a parent may result in feelings of anger, guilt, and depression. Psychological conflicts that existed between mothers and daughters may be rekindled; problems that already existed between spouses may intensify as a result of the additional demands on time and emotions. When caregivers enter into a relationship with the relative's physician, additional conflicts may ensue, as the caregiver and the physician may hold an opinion contrary to the relative's (Haug: 1994).

As difficult as this situation is for healthy caregivers, caregivers who have disabilities or chronic conditions may feel that they are neglecting their parents if they do not help with the provision of care and services. While they may hold unrealistic expectations for themselves, they may feel guilty for not being able to devote time or energy to their parents. Hiring a case manager may be the best solution. Some case managers are in private practice, while others may be located at publicly funded agencies on aging. Case managers evaluate the person's needs, recommend appropriate services, and follow up to ensure that the services are being provided.

To relieve the burden on family members, many state departments on aging have programs that provide assistance to elders living at home who need additional care. Financial assistance for these programs is also available. Employment of a home health aide alleviates some of the burdens placed on the family caregiver. Every state has a department on aging which funds agencies throughout the state to implement its programs.

Other options that may prove useful to the family caregiver include support groups of family members in similar situations. Many of the national voluntary organizations that are dedicated to a single disease or disability sponsor these support groups. Employers, recognizing the growing needs of their employees in the area of eldercare, have begun to provide assistance as well. Flexible time schedules, allowing employees to use pre-tax income for medical assistance for relatives, information and referral services, and on-site adult day care are a few of the programs that are now available at places of employment.

The Family and Medical Leave Act of 1993 (P.L. 103-3) enables eligible employees to take unpaid leave from work to care for sick relatives without forfeiting their jobs or their benefits (see Chapter 2, "Laws that Affect Elders with Disabilities" for a more detailed description of this act).

The National Family Caregiver Support Program (NFCSP) was established through the Older Americans Act Amendments of 2000 (P.L. 106-501). It is designed to help family members provide care for elders at home (see Chapter 2, "Laws that Affect Elders with Disabilities" for a more detailed description of this act).

COMPUTERS AND DISABILITIES

Both elders and family members can benefit from the use of personal computers. Public libraries, senior centers, and adult education programs offer computer training courses free or at low cost. Large monitors and software programs that enlarge the print size provide access to computer resources for elders with vision loss. Used alone, adapted computers enable individuals to perform tasks that would be otherwise inaccessible to them; retaining a job is just one major opportunity that computers offer to elders with disabilities. Using computers with online subscription services and the Internet, it is possible to communicate with people all over the world. This instant communication provides up-to-the-minute information about new developments and the opportunity to "chat" with individuals in similar situations. Many of these services are free, with the exception of telephone charges or subscription fees.

World Wide Web pages provide access to information from service agencies, professional societies, educational institutions, and commercial organizations, as well as individuals who have established their own pages. Web sites listed throughout this book provide links to a wide variety of disability resources.

A variety of formats is available to receive and exchange information. When you join a usenet group, you may read messages and respond to them as well as submit your own information and questions. In order to join a usenet group, your host computer must provide access. When you subscribe to a usenet group, you will automatically receive all new messages whenever you log on. If you decide to exchange messages with just one member, you may send mail directly to that individual's e-mail address.

Listserv enables you to receive information by sending a message to an e-mail address stating you would like to subscribe. You may add your own messages which may in turn generate responses from other members of a group. Protocol requires that you then summarize your responses and mail them to all other members of the listserv group.

PubMed is a web site that provides access to MEDLINE, a medical database that enables the user to perform searches of the medical literature by topic and author. PubMed is available over the Internet at no charge, directly from the National Library of Medicine, as are several other online databases. MEDLINE performs searches of major medical journals and provides both citations and abstracts of articles. After searching MEDLINE and reading abstracts of the articles on the web site, it is possible to order the articles. You may also find the articles at local libraries. If your library does not have the articles you want, ask the reference librarians to obtain them from other libraries. Be certain to ask the charge, as it may be less expensive for you to visit the other libraries yourself. Alternately, many medical school libraries, which are a good source of these articles, are open to the public.

CONCLUSION

Rehabilitation, independent living programs, and self-help groups are some of the options available at the local level that help elders with disabilities. When these local services are used in conjunction with the resources described in this book, elders may overcome the depression that often accompanies physical impairments and achieve the maximum possible level of independence.

REFERENCES

Administration on Aging
2001   A PROFILE OF OLDER AMERICANS 2001 Washington, DC:
       US Department of Health and Human Services
American Association of Retired Persons
1998   A PROFILE OF OLDER AMERICANS: 1998

American Geriatrics Society

1998 "The Management of Chronic Pain in Older Adults" JOURNAL OF THE AMERICAN GERIATRICS SOCIETY 46:5:635-651

Benedict, Robert C. and Mary L. Ganikos

1981 "Coming to Terms with Ageism in Rehabilitation" JOURNAL OF REHABILITATION 47 (October/November/December): 10-17

Bruce, Martha Livingston et al.

1994 "The Impact of Depressive Symptomatology on Physical Disability: MacArthur Studies of Successful Aging" AMERICAN JOURNAL OF PUBLIC HEALTH 84(November)11:1796-1799

Glass, Laurel E. and Holly H. Elliott

1992 "The Professionals Told Me What It Was, But That's Not Enough" SHHH JOURNAL (January/February):26-28

Greenblatt, Susan L.

1991 "What People with Vision Loss Need to Know" pp. 7-20 in Susan L. Greenblatt (ed.) MEETING THE NEEDS OF PEOPLE WITH VISION LOSS: A MULTIDISCIPLINARY PERSPECTIVE Lexington, MA: Resources for Rehabilitation

1988 "Physicians and Chronic Impairment: A Study of Ophthalmologists' Interactions with Visually Impaired and Blind Patients" SOCIAL SCIENCE AND MEDICINE 26:4:393-399

Haug, Marie R.

1994 "Elderly Patients, Caregivers, and Physicians: Theory and Research on Health Care Triads" JOURNAL OF HEALTH AND SOCIAL BEHAVIOR 35(March):1-12

Hollander, Laura-Lee

1982 "Normal Aging" pp. 1-39 in Martha Logigian (ed.) ADULT REHABILITATION: A TEAM APPROACH FOR THERAPISTS Boston, MA: Little Brown & Company

Madara, Edward
No DEVELOPING SELF-HELP GROUPS - GENERAL
date STEPS AND GUIDELINES FOR PROFESSIONALS Denville,
NJ: New Jersey Self-Help Clearinghouse

Manton, Kenneth G. and Beth J. Soldo
1992 "Disability and Mortality among the Oldest Old: Implications for Current and Future Health and Long-Term Care
Service Needs" pp. 199-250 in Richard M. Suzman et al.
(eds.) THE OLDEST OLD New York, NY: Oxford University
Press

McNeil, Jack
2001 AMERICANS WITH DISABILITIES 1997: CURRENT POPULA-
TION REPORTS P70-73 Washington, DC: U.S. Census
Bureau

Norburn, Jean E. et al.
1995 "Self-Care and Assistance From Others in Coping With
Functional Status Limitations Among a National Sample of
Older Adults" JOURNAL OF GERONTOLOGY
50B(No.2):S101-109

Rodin, Judith
1989 "Sense of Control: Potentials for Intervention" ANNALS
OF THE AMERICAN ACADEMY OF POLITICAL AND SOCIAL
SCIENCE 503(May):29-42

Taylor, Kenya S.
1991 "Survey Finds Physicians Often Fail to Refer Hearing-
Impaired Elderly" THE HEARING JOURNAL 44(November)11:36-39

Tinetti, Mary E. and Lynda Powell
1993 "Fear of Falling and Low Self-Efficacy: A Cause of
Dependency in Elderly Persons" JOURNALS OF
GERONTOLOGY Vol. 48(Special Issue):35-38

U.S. Department of Health and Human Services
1991 AGING IN AMERICA TRENDS AND PROJECTIONS DHHS
Publication No. (FCoA) 91-28001

ORGANIZATIONS

AARP
formerly American Association of Retired Persons
601 E Street, NW
Washington DC 20049
(800) 424-3410   www.aarp.org

A membership organization that advocates on behalf of elders. Administers insurance and investment programs and offers a discount pharmacy service.   Membership, $12.50, includes "AARP News Bulletin," "My Generation" (for members age 50-55), and "Modern Maturity" (for members over age 55).

ADMINISTRATION ON AGING (AoA)
U.S. Department of Health and Human Services
200 Independence Avenue, SW
Washington, DC 20201
(202) 619-0724   www.aoa.gov

A federal agency that acts as an advocate for elders within the federal government. Administers grants, sponsors research, and prepares and disseminates information related to problems of elders. Provides technical assistance to state and area agencies on aging.

AGENCY FOR HEALTHCARE RESEARCH AND QUALITY (AHRQ)
2101 East Jefferson Street, Suite 501
Rockville, MD 20852
(301) 594-1364   www.ahrq.gov

A federal agency that funds research studies on effectiveness of medical treatments, economic aspects of health care policy, and quality of care.   Publishes monthly newsletter, "Research

Activities." FREE. Newsletter and reports also available on the web site.

ALLIANCE FOR AGING RESEARCH (AFAR)
2021 K Street, NW, Suite 305
Washington, DC 20006
(202) 293-2856   FAX (202) 785-8574
www.agingresearch.org

An organization that promotes increased federal research into health and the aging process; informs the public about current research findings; and holds conferences. Publishes online newsletter, "Living Longer and Loving It," quarterly. Produces numerous publications related to health issues affecting elders. Single copies, FREE. Also available on the web site.

AMERICAN GERIATRICS SOCIETY (AGS)
350 Fifth Avenue, Suite 801
New York, NY 10118
(800) 677-9944   (212) 308-1414
FAX (212) 832-8646   www.americangeriatrics.org

This professional organization for physicians and other health care professionals provides training and research opportunities. Membership, physicians, $215.00; other health care professionals, $195.00. Includes a subscription to the "Journal of the American Geriatrics Society" and the "AGS Newsletter."

AMERICAN SELF-HELP CLEARINGHOUSE
100 Hanover Avenue, Suite 202
Cedar Knolls, NJ 07927
(973) 326-6789   FAX (973) 326-9467
www.selfhelpgroups.org

Provides information and contacts for national self-help groups, information on model groups and individuals who are starting new networks, and state or local self-help clearinghouses.

AMERICAN SOCIETY ON AGING (ASA)
833 Market Street, Suite 511
San Francisco, CA 94103
(415) 974-9600   FAX (415) 974-0300
www.asaging.org

A multidisciplinary membership organization that provides education and training and sponsors networks of special interest groups. Membership fees vary.

CAREGIVERS CORNER
www.mayoclinic.com

This web site provides information on home adaptation, safety, advance directives, long term care, and other topics for caregivers of elders.

CAREPLANNER
www2.careplanner.org

Developed by the Centers for Medicare and Medicaid Services and Clinical Tools, Inc., this web site provides a tool that may help elders, families, and professionals make decisions about health, financial, personal, and caregiver issues. It may be used online and an individualized Advice Report will be generated. The questions may also be printed, answered, and entered into the computer at a later time and an individualized advice report will be sent.

CHILDREN OF AGING PARENTS (CAPS)
Woodbourne Office Campus, Suite 302A
1609 Woodbourne Road
Levittown, PA 19057
(800) 227-7294   (215) 945-6900
www.caps4caregivers.org

Helps caregivers find the appropriate care and support for elders as well as for themselves. A caregiver guide is available online. Sponsors a network of support groups for caregivers. Publishes a variety of training and resource materials for support groups and a bimonthly newsletter, "CAPSule." Membership, individuals, $20.00; professionals and organizations, $100.00.

CLINICALTRIALS.GOV
clinicaltrials.gov

This confidential web site has information on more than 4,000 Federal and private medical studies. Lists location of clinical trials, design and purpose, criteria for participation, information about the disease and treatment being studied, and links to personnel who are recruiting participants. Also available at www.nlm.nih.gov

COMBINED HEALTH INFORMATION DATABASE (CHID)
Ovid Technologies, Attn: CHID Database
333 7th Avenue
New York, NY 10001
(800) 950-2035   (212) 563-3006
chid.nih.gov

A federally sponsored database that includes bibliographic citations and abstracts from journals, reports, books, and patient education brochures. FREE

DEPARTMENT OF VETERANS AFFAIRS (VA)
(800) 827-1000   www.va.gov

This nationwide toll-free number connects veterans with the VA regional office in their vicinity.

DISABILITY.GOV
www.disability.gov

This web site provides links to a wide variety of information and resources of the federal government that are related to disability.

DISABILITYRESOURCES.ORG
Disability Resources, Inc.
Dept. IN
4 Glatter Lane
Centereach, NY 11720
(631) 585-0290 (V/FAX)
www.disabilityresources.org

The web site provides information about resources for independent living, including "The DRM Regional Resource Directory." Publishes "Disability Resources Monthly," $33.00. Available in standard print and audiocassette. FREE sample available on the web site.

ELDERCARE LOCATOR
National Association of Area Agencies on Aging (NAAAA)
(800) 677-1116   (202) 296-8130
www.eldercare.gov

A nationwide information and referral service that provides callers with the phone number for a local information and referral service, which in turn provides the name of a local agency that can help with their specific needs. FREE. Also available on the web site.

ELDERNET
1330 Beacon Street, Suite 268
Brookline, MA 02446
(617) 244-1774   www.eldernet.com

Developed by an attorney who specializes in issues that affect elders, this web site provides information and links related to health, housing, finances, laws, and retirement.

FEDERAL TRADE COMMISSION (FTC)
Bureau of Consumer Protection
600 Pennsylvania Avenue, NW
Washington, DC 20580
(877) 382-4357   (202) 382-4357
(202) 326-2502 (TTY)   FAX (202) 326-2572
www.ftc.gov

This federal agency is mandated to protect consumers against unfair, deceptive, or fraudulent practices, including advertising, marketing, and sales of over-the-counter drugs, health care goods, and services. Ten regional offices. To register complaints or comments about health claims, send e-mail to: health-claims@ftc.gov FREE publications list.

FIRST GOV FOR CONSUMERS
www.consumer.gov

This cooperative project of the Food and Drug Administration, Federal Trade Commission, Consumer Products Safety Commission, National Highway Transportation Safety Administration, and Securities and Exchange Commission offers consumer information on topics such as health and safety, money and credit, transportation, and food safety. Includes information on FDA warnings and alerts and information for elders.

FIRST GOV FOR SENIORS
www.seniors.gov

This web site provides information on topics such as consumer protection, health, legislation, retirement plans, travel and leisure, and seniors and computers.

FOUNDATION FOR HEALTH IN AGING
350 Fifth Avenue, Suite 801
New York, NY 10118
(800) 563-4916   (212) 755-6810
www.healthinaging.org

This foundation, sponsored by the American Geriatrics Society, focuses on public education and clinical research. The web site provides information on health issues related to elders.

GENERATIONS ON LINE
108 Ralston House
3615 Chestnut Street
Philadelphia, PA 19104
(215) 222-6400   www.generationsonline.com

This organization is dedicated to increasing Internet literacy among elders in order to enhance their lives. Provides software and support to senior centers, nursing homes, and libraries.

GERONTOLOGICAL SOCIETY OF AMERICA (GSA)
1030 15th Street, NW, Suite 250
Washington, DC 20005
(202) 842-1275   www.geron.org

A multidisciplinary membership organization for professionals with an interest in aging. Sponsors fellowship program in applied gerontology. Membership, $120.00, includes choice of two of three: "Journals of Gerontology," "The Gerontologist," and "Gerontology News."

HEALTHFINDER
www.healthfinder.gov

Sponsored by the federal government, this web site provides information about government agencies that are related to health, as well as online publications such as a medical dictionary.

HEALTHPAGES
www.thehealthpages.com

Provides articles on a wide variety of diseases and conditions. Also provides information on physicians and facilities that treat specific disorders in specified metropolitan areas.

HEALTHWEB
www.healthweb.org

This web site is operated by a consortium of university libraries. The site provides links to a variety of noncommercial health sites that have been evaluated by the librarians.

INFOAGING.ORG
American Federation for Aging Research (AFAR)
70 West 40th Street, 11th Floor
New York, NY 10018
(212) 703-9977   FAX (212) 997-0330
www.infoaging.org

This web site provides information on age-related diseases and conditions.

LIBRARIANS' INDEX TO THE INTERNET
lii.org

This searchable, annotated subject directory on Internet resources includes subjects such as disabilities, health, medicine, and seniors.

MEDICINENET
www.medicinenet.com

Sponsored by physicians, this web site provides information on diseases, procedures and tests, drugs, a medical dictionary, and links to other health sites.

MEDLINEPLUS: SENIORS' HEALTH
www.nlm.nih.gov/medlineplus/seniorshealthgeneral.html

This web site provides links to sites for general information about seniors' health, prevention and screening, specific conditions/aspects, law and policy, organizations, clinical trials, statistics, and research. Some information is available in Spanish. Provides links to MEDLINE research articles and related MEDLINEplus pages.

NATIONAL AGING INFORMATION CENTER (NAIC)
330 Independence Avenue, SW, Room 4656
Washington, DC 20201
(202) 619-7501   FAX (202) 401-7620
www.aoa.gov/naic

Provides information and statistics on aging to policy makers, service providers, and the public. FREE publications list. Also available on the web site.   Web site also provides links to caregiver resources.

NATIONAL ALLIANCE FOR CAREGIVING
4720 Montgomery Lane, Suite 642
Bethesda, MD 20814
(301) 718-8444   FAX (301) 652-7711
www.caregiving.org

An alliance of several national groups concerned with issues of aging, this organization supports research, outreach programs, and a clearinghouse of resources. The AXA Foundation Family Care Resource Connection database, available on the web site, allows family caregivers to search for information on topics such as medical conditions, hands-on caregiving skills, legal and financial information, coping with caregiving, and community resources. Entries are rated for quality and usefulness.

NATIONAL ASSOCIATION FOR HOME CARE (NAHC)
228 7th Street, SE
Washington, DC 20003
(202) 547-7424   FAX (202) 547-3540
www.nahc.org

Trade association of home care and hospice organizations. Consumer education publications include "How to Choose a Home Care Provider," and "How to Choose a Home Care Agency." Single copies, FREE. Also available on the web site.

NATIONAL ASSOCIATION OF PROFESSIONAL GERIATRIC CARE MANAGERS
1604 North Country Club Road
Tucson, AZ 85716
(520) 881-8008   FAX (520) 325-7295
www.caremanager.org

An organization of professionals who provide counseling and case management for frail elders and their families. Members help plan for appropriate care and arrange to hire service providers. The "Find a Care Manager" database may be searched online.

NATIONAL FAMILY CAREGIVERS ASSOCIATION
10400 Connecticut Avenue, Suite 500
Kensington, MD 20895
(800) 896-3650   FAX (301) 942-2302
www.nfcacares.org

A membership organization for individuals who provide care for others at any stage of their lives or with any disease or disability. Maintains an information clearinghouse. Membership, U.S. family caregivers, FREE; other individuals, $20.00; professionals, $40.00; nonprofit organizations, $60.00; and group medical practices, home health agencies, etc., $100.00. Membership includes quarterly newsletter, "Take Care!" which provides information and resources for family caregivers.

NATIONAL HEALTH INFORMATION CENTER
Office of Disease Prevention and Health Promotion
PO Box 1133
Washington, DC 20013-1133
(800) 336-4797   In MD, (301) 565-4167
FAX (301) 984-4256   FAXBACK (301) 468-1204
nhic-nt.health.org

Maintains a database of health-related organizations and a library. Provides referrals related to health issues for both professionals and consumers. Publications enable individuals to locate information and resources in the federal government. FREE publications list; also available on the web site. Publications on the web site include "Federal Health Information Centers and Clearinghouses" with telephone numbers and web sites for federal health information and referral services by topic.

NATIONAL INSTITUTE ON AGING (NIA)
National Institutes of Health
Building 31
Bethesda, MD 20892
(301) 496-1752   www.nia.nih.gov

A federal agency that supports basic and clinical research on a broad range of issues that affect elders. Funds Older Americans Independence Centers, which test interventions to prevent or minimize functional impairments; Centers of Research on Applied Gerontology, which study topics such as disabling conditions, physical activity and fitness, and injury; and Geriatric Research and Training Centers. Professional and consumer information publications. FREE

NATIONAL INSTITUTES OF HEALTH INFORMATION
www.nih.gov/health

Provides a single access point to the National Institutes of Health, including their individual clearinghouses, publications, and the Combined Health Information Database. Provides information on hotlines, PubMed, clinical trials and drug information.

NATIONAL LIBRARY OF MEDICINE (NLM)
8600 Rockville Pike
Building 38, Room 2S-10
Bethesda, MD 20894
(888) 346-3656   (301) 594-5983
www.ncbi.nlm.nih.gov/PubMed

Operates PubMed, a web site which provides access to MEDLINE, a computerized database that provides access to articles in major medical journals from around the world. Users may search for a specific health related topic and receive citations and abstracts of articles. Available directly through NLM's web site and at most medical, public, and university libraries.

NATIONAL REHABILITATION INFORMATION CENTER (NARIC)
4200 Forbes Boulevard, Suite 202
Lanham, MD 20706
(800) 346-2742   (301) 459-5900
www.naric.com

A federally funded center that responds to telephone and mail inquiries about disabilities and support services. Maintains REHABDATA, a database with publications and research references. Some NARIC publications are available on the web site.

NATIONAL SELF-HELP CLEARINGHOUSE
Graduate School and University Center of the City University of New York
365 5th Avenue, Suite 3300
New York, NY 10016
(212) 817-1822   www.selfhelpweb.org

Makes referrals to local self-help groups.

NIH SENIOR HEALTH
nihseniorhealth.gov

This web site provides information on topics such as Alzheimer's Disease, caregiving, and exercise for older adults. Includes videos that may be viewed online.

RESOURCES FOR REHABILITATION
22 Bonad Road
Winchester, MA 01890
(781) 368-9094   FAX (781) 368-9096
www.rfr.org

An organization that provides training and information to professionals who serve people with disabilities and to the public. Publications, training programs, program evaluations, and needs assessments.

SENIORNET
121 Second Street, 7th Floor
San Francisco, CA 94105
(800) 747-6848   (415) 495-4990
FAX (415) 495-3999   www.seniornet.org

Maintains network of SeniorNet Learning Centers across the U.S. which provide computer training to adults age 50 and over. Sells computer tutorials. Membership, $30.00, includes quarterly newsletter and discounts on products.

SPRY FOUNDATION
10 G Street, NE, Suite 600
Washington, DC 20002
(202) 216-0401   (202) 216-0779
www.spry.org

This foundation focuses on research and education that will help to achieve successful aging. Among its current projects, it is studying how elders obtain health information and how they make medical decisions.

UNITED WAY OF AMERICA (UWA)
701 North Fairfax Street
Alexandria, VA 22314
(800) 411-8929 to obtain telephone number of closest United Way office
(703) 836-7100   FAX (703) 683-7840
www.unitedway.org

An umbrella organization of local human service organizations. National office will direct callers to the local United Way, which in turn will provide referral to a specific local service agency.

VISITING NURSE ASSOCIATIONS OF AMERICA (VNAA)
11 Beacon Street, Suite 910
Boston, MA 02108
(617) 523-4042   FAX (617) 227-4843
www.vnaa.org

Provides referrals to local Visiting Nurse Associations which offer services such as skilled nursing care, hospice care, home health aides, social work and counseling services, and Meals on Wheels. "Find a VNA" is available online only.

WELL SPOUSE FOUNDATION
30 East 40th Street, Suite PH
New York, NY 10016
(800) 838-0879   (212) 685-8815
FAX (212) 685-8676   www.wellspouse.org

A network of support groups that provide emotional support to husbands, wives, and partners of people who are chronically ill. Membership, individuals, $25.00; professionals, $50.00; includes bimonthly newsletter, "Mainstay." Publishes pamphlets discussing "Guilt," "Anger," "Isolation," and "Looking Ahead." $1.50 each; $5.00 per set.

PUBLICATIONS AND TAPES

AGELINE
AARP
formerly American Association of Retired Persons
601 E Street, NW
Washington DC 20049
(800) 424-3410   www.research.aarp.org/ageline

A bibliographic database that provides citations and abstracts on social, psychological, economic, political, and health issues related to aging. Available online and on CD-ROM.

AGING AND REHABILITATION II
Stanley J. Brody and L. Gregory Pawlson (eds.)
Springer Publishing Company, New York, NY

A collection of articles written by a multidisciplinary group of authors who suggest practical interventions for common problems, including environmental adaptations and nutrition therapy. Out of print

AMERICAN GERIATRICS SOCIETY'S COMPLETE GUIDE TO AGING AND HEALTH
by Mark E. Williams
American Geriatrics Society (AGS)
350 Fifth Avenue, Suite 801
New York, NY 10118
(800) 677-9944   (212) 308-1414
FAX (212) 832-8646   www.americangeriatrics.org

A medical reference for elders and caregivers, with information on the aging process, making medical decisions, and strategies for preventing illness. $26.00

THE CAREGIVER'S GUIDE: HELPING ELDERLY RELATIVES COPE WITH HEALTH AND SAFETY PROBLEMS
by Caroline Rob and Janet Reynolds
Houghton Mifflin Company
181 Ballardvale Street
Wilmington, MA 01887
(800) 225-3362   FAX (800) 634-7568
www.hmco.com

This book covers a wide range of health problems, including cancer, pain, pneumonia, skin disease, digestive problems, and sleep disorders. $15.00

CAREGIVER'S HANDBOOK: A COMPLETE GUIDE TO HOME HEALTH CARE
by Visiting Nurse Associations of America
Dorling Kindersley
375 Hudson Street
New York, NY 10014
(877) 342-5357   (212) 213-4800
www.dk.com

This book offers practical advice, emotional support, and information for daily caregiving. Includes illustrated techniques, information on benefits, patient's bill of rights, and a glossary. $14.95

CAREGIVING: THE SPIRITUAL JOURNEY OF LOVE, LOSS AND RENEWAL
by Beth Witrogen McLeod
John Wiley and Sons
Consumer Center
10475 Crosspoint Boulevard
Indianapolis, IN 46256
(877) 762-2974   FAX (800) 597-3299
www.wiley.com

This book uses caregiver stories, interviews, and literary references to provide strategies for coping with the stress of caring for loved ones. It discusses topics such as women and caregiving, emotional stresses, end-of-life concerns, and recovery from loss. $14.95

CARING FOR YOURSELF WHILE CARING FOR OTHERS: SURVIVAL AND RENEWAL
by Lawrence M. Brammer
Vantage Press
516 West 34th Street
New York, NY 10001
(800) 882-3273   (212) 736-1767
FAX (212) 736-2273   www.vantagepress.com

This book discusses coping and survival strategies and suggests how to face difficult feelings. Provides community resources and reading lists. $14.95

CHOOSING MEDICAL CARE IN OLD AGE: WHAT KIND, HOW MUCH, WHEN TO STOP
by Muriel R. Gillick
Harvard University Press
79 Garden Street
Cambridge, MA 02138
(800) 405-1619   (617) 495-2480
FAX (800) 406-9145   www.hup.harvard.edu

Written by a geriatrician, this book discusses the issues that face elders in making choices for medical care, whether they are frail, robust, terminally ill, or if others must make choices for them. Hardcover, $20.95; softcover, $14.95.

COMING HOME: BASIC INFORMATION FOR THE HOME CAREGIVER
Terra Nova Films
9848 South Winchester Avenue
Chicago, IL 60643
(800) 779-8491   (773) 881-8491
FAX (773) 881-3368   www.terranova.org

This videotape reviews five basic caregiving concerns: moving and transfer, infection control, nutrition, stress, and talking with the doctor. 51 minutes. Purchase, $129.00; one week rental, $45.00.

DISABILITY FUNDING NEWS
CD Publications
8204 Fenton Street
Silver Spring, MD 20910
(800) 666-6380   (301) 588-6380
FAX (301) 588-6385
www.cdpublications.com/cdpubs

This semimonthly publication contains information about funding opportunities from the federal government and private foundations. $339.00

ELDERCARE AT HOME
by Peter S. Houts and Laurence Z. Rubenstein (eds.)
Foundation for Health in Aging
American Geriatrics Society (AGS)
350 Fifth Avenue, Suite 801
New York, NY 10118
(800) 563-4916   (212) 755-6810
www.healthinaging.org

This online manual provides information for caregivers on physical problems such as pain, incontinence, and sleep; mental and social problems such as depression, communication, memory loss, and dementia; and managing care, including daily living issues, advance directives, choosing a nursing home, and community resources. Chapters may be downloaded at no charge.

HELPING YOURSELF HELP OTHERS: A BOOK FOR CAREGIVERS
by Rosalynn Carter with Susan K. Golant
Random House, Order Department
400 Hahn Road, PO Box 100
Westminster, MD 21157
(800) 733-3000   www.randomhouse.com

This book focuses on family caregivers, offering suggestions for everyday problems such as physical and emotional needs, isolation, burnout, and dealing with professional caregivers. Lists of organizations, books, and resources included. $14.00

HOW TO CARE FOR AGING PARENTS
by Virginia Morris
Workman Publishing Company, Inc.
708 Broadway
New York, NY 10003
(800) 722-7202   (212) 254-5900
FAX (212) 254-8098   www.workman.com

This guide provides practical information for caregivers and those they are caring for. Includes chapters on caregiver resources, daily living activities, finances, legal issues, housing, medical care and conditions, and death and grieving. $15.95

LIFELINES: LIVING LONGER, GROWING FRAIL, TAKING HEART
by Muriel Gillick
W. W. Norton & Company
800 Keystone Industrial Park
Scranton, PA 18512
(800) 223-2588   (717) 346-2029
FAX (800) 458-6515   www.wwnorton.com

This book describes the challenges faced by four elders who have grown progressively frail. It suggests strategies for prevention of frailty in physical, psychological, cognitive, and social areas. $25.95

MAKING WISE MEDICAL DECISIONS: HOW TO GET THE INFORMATION YOU NEED
Resources for Rehabilitation
22 Bonad Road
Winchester, MA 01890
(781) 368-9094   FAX (781) 368-9096
www.rfr.org

This book includes information about where to go and what to read in order to make informed, rational, medical decisions. It describes how to obtain relevant health information and evaluate medical tests and procedures, health care providers, and health facilities. Includes chapters on special issues facing elders and people with chronic illnesses and disabilities. $42.95. (See last page of this book for order form.)

NATIONAL INSTITUTE ON AGING PUBLICATIONS LIST
NIA Information Center
PO Box 8057
Gaithersburg, MD 20898-8057
(800) 222-2225
www.nia.nih.gov/health/orderinfo.htm

Describes the publications that are available from NIA for professionals and the public. FREE. Publishes AGE PAGE, a series of fact sheets about a variety of health and safety issues related to aging, such as "Considering Surgery?" "Hospital Hints," and "Who's Who in Health Care." LARGE PRINT. FREE. Also available on the web site.

THE NEW OURSELVES GROWING OLDER
by Paula B. Doress-Worters and Diana Laskin Siegal
Simon and Schuster
100 Front Street
Riverside, NJ 08075
(888) 866-6631   FAX (800) 943-9831
www.simonsays.com

This book provides information and resources for midlife and older women. Topics include aging, sexuality, disabilities, health care, employment, housing, and finances. $20.00

ON OUR OWN: INDEPENDENT LIVING FOR OLDER PERSONS
by Ursula A. Falk
Prometheus Books
59 John Glenn Drive
Amherst, NY 14228
(800) 421-0351   www.prometheusbooks.com

This book discusses the emotional aspects of aging alone, community resources, safety, family relationships, and financial issues. $21.00. Also available on 4-track audiocassette from National Library Service for the Blind and Physically Handicapped regional libraries, RC 31678. FREE

THE RESOURCE DIRECTORY FOR OLDER PEOPLE
National Institute on Aging Information Center
PO Box 8057
Gaithersburg, MD 20898-8057
(800) 222-2225   (800) 222-4225 (TTY)
(301) 587-2528
www.nia.nih.gov/health

This directory lists federal, state, and private organizations that work with older adults. Includes lists of state agencies on aging and long term care ombudsman programs. Single copy, FREE. Also available on the web site.

THE SELF-HELP SOURCEBOOK ONLINE
American Self-Help Clearinghouse
100 Hanover Avenue, Suite 202
Cedar Knolls, NJ 07927
(973) 326-6789   FAX (973) 326-9467
www.selfhelpgroups.org

This online database provides information on national and model self-help groups, online mutual help groups and networks, and self-help clearinghouses. Includes ideas on starting self-help groups and opportunities to link with others to develop new groups.

WHO CARES: SOURCES OF INFORMATION ABOUT HEALTH CARE PRODUCTS AND SERVICES
Bureau of Consumer Protection, Federal Trade Commission
600 Pennsylvania Avenue, NW
Washington, DC 20580
(877) 382-4357   (202) 382-4357
(202) 326-2502 (TTY)   FAX (202) 326-2572
www.ftc.gov

This booklet lists federal, state, and private resources for information on subjects such as hearing aids, prescription drugs, nursing facilities, and medical treatments. FREE

Chapter 2
LAWS THAT AFFECT ELDERS WITH DISABILITIES

Laws that affect elders with disabilities cover a wide range of issues, including health care, financial benefits, housing, rehabilitation, civil rights, transportation, access to public buildings, and employment. For those who are not specialists in the law, it is sometimes difficult to keep abreast of the laws and their amendments. At the same time, elders with disabilities may be able to continue living independently if they are aware of their rights and know how to locate the proper equipment and professional services. In many instances, government programs provide financial assistance for these needs.

The REHABILITATION ACT of 1973 (P.L. 93-112) and its amendments are the centerpieces of federal law related to rehabilitation. States must submit a vocational rehabilitation plan to the Rehabilitation Services Administration, indicating how the designated state agency will provide vocational training, counseling, and diagnostic and evaluation services required by the law. The "Client Assistance Program" (P.L. 98-221) authorizes states to inform clients and other persons with disabilities about all available benefits under the Act and to assist them in obtaining all remedies due under the law. "Comprehensive Services for Independent Living" (P.L. 95-602) expands rehabilitation services to individuals with severe disabilities, regardless of their vocational potential, making services available to many elders who are no longer in the work force. The Act broadly defines services as any "service that will enhance the ability of a handicapped individual to live independently or function within his family and community..." These services may include counseling, job placement, housing, funds to make the home accessible, funds for prosthetic devices, attendant care, and recreational activities. The Rehabilitation Act Amendments of 1992 (P.L. 102-569) establish state rehabilitation advisory councils composed of representatives of independent living councils, parents of children with disabilities, vocational rehabilitation professionals, and business; the role of these councils is to advise state vocational rehabilitation agencies and to prepare an annual report for the governor. Each state agency was required to establish performance and evaluation standards by September 30, 1994. The amendments also establish a National Commission on Rehabilitation Services to study the quality and adequacy of rehabilitation services provided by the states.

SUPPLEMENTARY SECURITY INCOME (SSI) is a federal minimum income maintenance program for elders and individuals who are blind or disabled and who meet a test of financial need. Monthly SOCIAL SECURITY DISABILITY INSURANCE (SSDI) benefits are available to individuals with disabilities and their dependents. To be eligible, individuals with disabilities must have paid Social Security taxes for a specified number of years (dependent upon the applicant's age); must not be working; and must be declared medically disabled by the state disability determination service or through an appeals process. The disability must be expected to last at least 12 months or to result in death. Individuals who are blind and age 55 to 65 may receive monthly benefits if they are unable to carry out the work (or similar work) that they did before age 55 or becoming blind, whichever is later. Individuals who have received SSDI for two consecutive years are eligible for MEDICARE, a federal health insurance program for people 65 or over, which may cover some of the necessary outpatient therapy or supplies discussed in this book. However, MEDICARE does not cover eyeglasses, low vision aids, or hearing aids. At the time this book went to press, Congress was debating legislation that would authorize Medicare to provide coverage for prescription drugs.

MEDICAID is a health insurance plan for individuals whose income is below a set level. MEDICAID is a joint federal/state venture, with many of the policies set at the state level. Therefore, payments for prosthetics or rehabilitation equipment vary greatly from state to state.

The FAMILY AND MEDICAL LEAVE ACT of 1993 (P.L.103-3) requires employers with 50 or more employees at a worksite or within 75 miles of a worksite to permit eligible employees 12 workweeks of unpaid leave during a 12 month period in order to care for a spouse, son or daughter, or parent who has a serious health condition. During this period of leave, the employer must continue to provide group health benefits for the employee under the same conditions as the employee would have received while working. Upon return from leave, the employee must be restored to the same position he or she had prior to the leave or to a position with equivalent pay, benefits, and conditions of employment. Special regulations apply to employees of school systems and private schools and employees of the federal civil service.

The TELECOMMUNICATIONS ACT of 1996 (P.L. 104-104) has several sections that apply to individuals with disabilities. Section 254 redefines "universal service" to include schools, health facilities, and libraries, and requires that the Federal Communications Commission (FCC) work with state governments to determine what services must be made universally available and what is considered "affordable." Section 255 requires that telecommunication equipment manufacturers and service providers be accessible to all individuals with disabilities, "if readily achievable." Section 713 requires that video services be accessible to individuals with hearing impairments via closed captioning and to individuals with visual impairments via descriptive video services. Section 706 requires that the FCC encourage the development of advanced telecommunications technology that provides equal access for individuals with disabilities, especially school children. The FCC is authorized to establish regulations and time tables for implementing these sections.

The TECHNOLOGY-RELATED ASSISTANCE FOR IN-DIVIDUALS WITH DISABILITIES ACT AMENDMENTS OF 1994 (P.L. 103-218) strengthen the original Act, passed in 1988. The Act mandates state-wide programs for technology-related assistance to determine needs and resources; to provide technical assistance and information; and to develop demonstration and innovation projects, training programs, and public awareness programs. The amendments set priorities for consumer responsiveness, advocacy, systems change, and outreach to underrepresented populations such as the poor, individuals in rural areas, and minorities.

The federal government allows special tax credits for elders who are totally disabled and additional standard deductions for those who are legally blind. Internal Revenue Service publications that explain these benefits include Publication 554, "Older Americans' Tax Guide," Publication 907, "Tax Highlights for Persons with Disabilities," Publication 501, "Exemptions, Standard Deduction, and Filing Information," and Publication 524, "Credit for the Elderly or the Disabled." Some states allow extra personal exemptions for legal blindness on state income tax as well.

In 1990, the AMERICANS WITH DISABILITIES ACT (ADA) was passed. Considered the most important piece of civil rights legislation in recent years, the ADA (P.L. 101-336) increases the steps employers must take to accommodate employees with disabilities and requires that public accommodations, new buses and rail vehicles, and facilities be accessible. The major provisions of the ADA are as follows:

> • Title I prohibits discrimination against individuals with disabilities who are otherwise qualified for employment and requires that employers make "reasonable accommodations." "Reasonable accommodations" include making existing facilities accessible and job restructuring (e.g., reassignment to a vacant position, modification of equipment, training, provision of interpreters and readers). Employers are protected from "undue hardship" in complying with this provision; the financial situation of the employer and the size and type of business are considered when deter-

mining whether an accommodation would constitute "undue hardship." The provisions of this section apply to employers with 15 or more employees. (For a more detailed discussion of the employment aspects of the ADA, see "Meeting the Needs of Employees with Disabilities," described in "PUBLICATIONS AND TAPES" section below).

· Title II prohibits discrimination by public entities (i.e., local and state governments) and requires that individuals with disabilities be entitled to the same rights and benefits of public programs as other individuals. For example, local programs for elders may not discriminate against those elders who have low vision or other disabilities; they are entitled to receive the same benefits of the programs as elders who do not have disabilities.

· Title III requires that public accommodations, businesses, and services be accessible to individuals with disabilities. Public accommodations are broadly defined to include places such as hotels and motels, theatres, museums, schools, shopping centers and stores, banks, restaurants, and professional service providers' offices. Effective January 26, 1993, most new construction for public accommodations must be accessible to individuals with disabilities.

· Requires that bus and railroad transportation systems address the needs of individuals with disabilities by purchasing adapted equipment, modifying facilities, and providing special transportation services that are comparable to regular transportation services.

· Title IV mandates that telephone companies provide relay services 24 hours a day, 7 days a week for individuals with hearing or speech impairments. Relay services enable individuals who have text telephones (TTY) or another computer device that is capable of communicating across telephone lines to communicate with individuals who do not have such devices.

In the years that have elapsed since the passage of the ADA, many court cases have resulted in clarifying and restricting the law's implementation.

For example, in 1999, the Supreme Court ruled in Olmstead, Commissioner, Georgia Department of Human Resources, et al. v. L.C. et al. that the ADA requires community placement instead of institutionalization whenever possible. The case was brought by two women who were both mentally retarded and mentally ill. Both had lived in state mental institutions for many years. Now their mental health professionals were recommending that they be placed in community-based treatment, but the state refused, saying it was more cost effective to keep the women hospitalized. The Supreme Court rejected the state's argument, citing Congress's intent that isolation and segregation were discrimination per se, and returned the case to the lower level court to determine appropriate relief. As a result of the Olmstead ruling, governments must place individuals in the community rather than in institutions whenever possible. This includes elders, who are often placed in nursing homes when supplemental in-home services could allow them to remain in their own homes.

Copies of the ADA are available from Senators and Representatives. (In addition, many private agencies that work with individuals with disabilities have copies of the ADA available for distribution to the public.) Agencies charged with formulating regulations and standards include the Architectural and Transportation Barriers Compliance Board, the Department of Transportation, the Equal Employment Opportunity Commission, the Federal Communications Commission, and the Attorney General. The Office of the Americans with Disabilities Act within the Department of Justice is responsible for enforcing the ADA. Regulations for enforcing individual sections of the act are available from the federal agencies charged with promulgating them and in the "Federal Register" (see "PUBLICATIONS" section below).

The FAIR HOUSING AMENDMENTS ACT OF 1988 (P.L. 100-430) prohibits discrimination in housing against individuals with disabilities and families with children. It provides tenants with disabilities the legal right to make modifications to rental housing at their own expense in order to meet their needs. However, the residence must be restored to its original condition "within reason" when the tenant moves. Multifamily dwellings of four or more units first occupied after March 13, 1991 must be accessible to individuals with disabilities.

Section 202 of the HOUSING AND COMMUNITY DEVELOPMENT ACT of 1987, Direct Loan Program for Housing for the Elderly or Handicapped, provides loans to nonprofit organizations to sponsor development of housing for elders and persons with disabilities, including units eligible for Section 8 rent subsidies. In 2000, HUD released the final rule that allows individuals and families to use Section 8 vouchers for home ownership. Public housing authorities who participate in the Homeownership Program can allow individuals and families to convert current Section 8 vouchers from rental to mortgage supplements and allow individuals and families who are eligible in the future to choose between mortgage and rental subsidies. The HOUSING AND COMMUNITY DEVELOPMENT ACT of 1992 permits owners of such housing projects to favor elderly tenants over those with disabilities who are not elders.

Section 801 of the NATIONAL AFFORDABLE HOUSING ACT of 1990, Supportive Housing for the Elderly, provides funds for nonprofit organizations to expand the supportive housing projects designed to meet the needs of elders. These supportive services may include meal service, housekeeping assistance, personal assistance, and transportation. Section 811, Supportive Housing for People with Disabilities, enables nonprofit organizations to develop group homes, independent living facilities, and intermediate care facilities licensed by state Medicaid agencies. Applications are available from Department of Housing and Urban Development (HUD) field offices.

The Rural Housing Service of the U.S. Department of Agriculture offers a variety of homeownership programs for individuals who are elderly, disabled, or low-income and who live in rural areas. These programs include direct loan and loan guarantees, home repair loan and grants, and rental assistance (see "ORGANIZATIONS" section below). Fannie Mae, a private company, offers HomeChoice, Community Living, and Retrofitting mortgages that make homeownership and home modifications possible for individuals with disabilities or who have family members with disabilities living with them (see "ORGANIZATIONS" section below).

Individuals who feel that they have been discriminated against may file complaints with HUD or a state or local fair housing agency, or they may file a civil suit.

In addition to the programs mandated for individuals with disabilities noted above, the OLDER AMERICANS ACT (P.L. 89-73) requires that each state office designated to serve elders submit a plan to the Commissioner of the Administration on Aging. This plan must discuss the development of joint programs with the state agency primarily responsible for serving people with disabilities in order to meet the needs of elders with disabilities. The Act also requires that legal services be provided to elders and that each state employ a legal services developer to ensure that elders receive these services. Such services could include representing clients in obtaining Social Security benefits and providing legal counseling. In 1992, amendments to the Older Americans Act established the Vulnerable Elders Rights Protection Program, designed to protect elders who are at risk for abuse due to physical or mental disabilities, financial status, social isolation, or limited education. Advocacy programs such as the Long-Term Care Ombudsman Program and programs for prevention of elder abuse, neglect, and exploitation are now in place. The Older Americans Act Amendments of 2000 (P.L. 106-501) included funding for the National Family Caregiver Support Program. It is designed to assist caregivers through information and assistance, counseling, support groups and training, respite services, and supplemental services. More than $141 million in grants were made to states for fiscal year 2002.

States may use Medicaid funds to compensate informal caregivers such as family members of the Medicaid beneficiary, with the exception of the individual who is legally responsible for that individual's care, i.e., the spouse, unless there are exceptional circumstances. Federal Medicaid policy allows the individual states to decide the circumstances under which family members are compensated.

All states and many local governments have adopted their own laws regarding accessibility. Information about these laws may be obtained from the state or local office serving people with disabilities. In many areas, special legal services for elders are available, often with fees on a sliding scale. The local bar association and law schools are good sources for this information. Some lawyers specialize in the legal needs of people with disabilities and of elders.

ORGANIZATIONS

ABA LAW INFO
www.abalawinfo.org

This web site offers a link to legal issues that affect the family and elders. Includes information on topics such as the rights of older Americans and laws and programs affecting elders. Publications may be downloaded at no charge.

ADMINISTRATION ON AGING (AoA)
U.S. Department of Health and Human Services
200 Independence Avenue, SW
Washington, DC 20201
(202) 619-0724   www.aoa.gov

Responsible for carrying out the provisions of the Older Americans Act and acts as an advocate for elders within the federal government. Funds several Senior Legal Assistance Programs throughout the country, which offer services such as Senior Legal Hotlines.

ARCHITECTURAL AND TRANSPORTATION BARRIERS COMPLIANCE BOARD (ATBCB)
1331 F Street, NW, Suite 1000
Washington, DC 20004
(800) 872-2253   (800) 993-2822 (TTY)
(202) 272-0080   (202) 272-0082 (TTY)
FAX (202) 272-0081   www.access-board.gov

A federal agency charged with developing standards for accessibility in federal facilities, public accommodations, and transportation facilities as required by the Americans with Disabilities Act and other federal laws. Provides technical assistance, sponsors research, and distributes publications. Publishes a quarterly newsletter, "Access America." Publications available in standard print, alternate formats, and on the web site. FREE

CENTERS FOR MEDICARE AND MEDICAID SERVICES (CMS)
formerly Health Care Financing Administration (HCFA)
7500 Security Boulevard
Baltimore, MD 21244
(800) 633-4227   (410) 786-3000
cms.hhs.gov

CMS is the federal agency that administers Medicare and Medicaid. Current Medicare regulations are available on the web site, as are many publications, including those about health care plans. Links to sites such as Medicare Health Plan Compare and Medigap Compare.

CLEARINGHOUSE ON DISABILITY INFORMATION
Office of Special Education and Rehabilitative Services (OSERS)
U.S. Department of Education
400 Maryland Avenue, SW
Washington, DC 20202
(800) 872-5327   (800) 437-0833 (TTY)
(202) 205-8241   FAX (202)) 401-0689
www.ed.gov/offices/OSERS

Responds to inquiries about federal legislation and programs for people with disabilities and makes referrals.

CLIENT ASSISTANCE PROGRAM (CAP)
U.S. Department of Education
Rehabilitation Services Administration
330 C Street, SW, Switzer Building, Room 3223
Washington, DC 20202
(202) 205-9315

Established by the Rehabilitation Act of 1973, as amended, CAP provides information and advocacy for individuals with disabilities served under the Act and Title I of the Americans with Disabilities Act. Assistance is also provided to facilitate employment.

COMMISSION ON LEGAL PROBLEMS OF THE ELDERLY
American Bar Association (ABA)
740 15th Street, NW, 9th Floor
Washington, DC 20005
(202) 662-8690   FAX (202) 662-8698
www.abanet.org/elderly

A multidisciplinary group that studies issues such as disability, health care, housing, and social security. Produces a variety of publications. Provides state listings of organizations funded under the Older Americans Act and other organizations that specialize in laws affecting elders. Single state profile, FREE; multiple copies or multiple state profiles, $1.00 each. Quarterly newsletter, "Bifocal," $35.00.

DISABILITY RIGHTS EDUCATION AND DEFENSE FUND (DREDF)
2212 6th Street
Berkeley, CA 94710
(510) 644-2555 (V/TTY)   FAX (510) 841-8645
www.dredf.org

Provides technical assistance, information, and referrals on laws and rights; provides legal representation to people with disabilities in both individual and class action cases; trains law students, parents, and legislators. ADA Hotline [(800)-466-4232 (V/TTY)] provides information on the Americans with Disabilities Act. Quarterly newsletter, "Disability Rights News," available in standard print, alternate formats, and on the web site. FREE

DISABILITY RIGHTS SECTION

U.S. Department of Justice, Civil Rights Division
950 Pennsylvania Avenue, NW
Washington, DC 20530
(800) 514-0301   (800) 514-0383 (TTY)
FAX (202) 307-1198
www.usdoj.gov/crt/ada/adahom1.htm

Responsible for enforcing Titles II and III of the Americans with Disabilities Act. Copies of its regulations are available in standard print, alternate formats, and on the web site. Callers may request publications, obtain technical assistance, and speak to an ADA specialist.

ELDERNET

1330 Beacon Street, Suite 268
Brookline, MA 02446
(617) 244-1774   www.eldernet.com

Developed by an attorney who specializes in issues that affect elders, this web site provides information and links related to health, housing, finances, laws, and retirement.

EQUAL EMPLOYMENT OPPORTUNITY COMMISSION (EEOC)

1801 L Street, NW, 10th floor
Washington, DC 20507
(800) 669-3362 to order publications
(800) 669-4000 to speak to an investigator
(800) 800-3302 (TTY)
In the Washington, DC metropolitan area, (202) 275-7377
(202) 275-7518 (TTY)   www.eeoc.gov

Responsible for promulgating and enforcing regulations for the employment section of the ADA. Copies of its regulations are available in standard print and alternate formats.

FANNIE MAE
(800) 732-6643   www.fanniemae.com

This private company offers mortgage products designed to help individuals with disabilities attain home ownership. Publishes "A Home of Your Own Guide," for housing educators and counselors who work with individuals with disabilities, available through the Fannie Mae Distribution Center, (800) 471-5554. FREE. Also available on the web site.

FEDERAL COMMUNICATIONS COMMISSION (FCC)
445 12th Street, SW
Washington, DC 20554
(888) 225-5322   (888) 835-5322 (TTY)
(202) 418-0190   (202) 418-2555 (TTY)
www.fcc.gov

Responsible for developing regulations for telecommunication issues related to federal laws, including the ADA and the Telecommunications Act of 1996.

INTERNAL REVENUE SERVICE (IRS)
(800) 829-1040   (800) 829-4059 (TTY)
www.irs.gov

The IRS provides technical assistance about tax credits and deductions related to accommodations for disabilities. To receive Publication 554, "Older Americans' Tax Guide," Publication 501, "Exemptions, Standard Deduction, and Filing Information;" Publication 907, "Tax Highlights for Persons with Disabilities;" and Publication 524, "Credit for the Elderly or the Disabled," call (800) 829-3676; (800) 829-4059 (TTY). These publications are available on the web site.

NATIONAL ACADEMY OF ELDER LAW ATTORNEYS
1604 North Country Club Road
Tucson, AZ 85716
(520) 881-4005   FAX (520) 325-7925
www.naela.com

A membership organization of attorneys who specialize in legal problems of elders. Publishes "Questions and Answers When Looking for an Elder Law Attorney," FREE. Also available on the web site. "A National Listing of Elder Law Attorneys," by geographic area and specialty, is also available on the web site.

NATIONAL COUNCIL ON DISABILITY (NCD)
1331 F Street, NW, Suite 850
Washington, DC 20004
(202) 272-2004   (202) 272-2074 (TTY)
FAX (202) 272-2022   www.ncd.gov

An independent federal agency mandated to study and make recommendations about public policy for people with disabilities. Holds regular meetings and hearings in various locations around the country. Publishes monthly newsletter, "NCD Bulletin," available in standard print, alternate formats, and on the web site. FREE

NOLO LAW FOR ALL
Nolo Press
950 Parker Street
Berkeley, CA 94710
(800) 992-6656   (510) 549-1976
FAX (800) 645-0895   www.nolo.com

This web site provides information on legal topics, updates legislation and court decisions, and features articles from "Nolo News." FREE publications catalogue.

OFFICE FOR CIVIL RIGHTS
U.S. Department of Health and Human Services
200 Independence Avenue, SW
Washington, DC 20201
(877) 696-6775   (202) 619-0700
(202) 863-0101 (TTY)   FAX (202) 619-3818
www.hhs.gov

Responsible for enforcing laws and regulations that protect the rights of individuals seeking medical and social services in institutions that receive federal financial assistance. Individuals who feel their rights have been violated may file a complaint with one of the ten regional offices located throughout the country. Calling (800) 368-1019 connects you with the regional office closest to you.

OFFICE OF CIVIL RIGHTS
Federal Transit Administration
400 7th Street, NW, Room 9102
Washington, DC 20590
(202) 366-3472   FAX (202) 366-3475
www.fta.dot.gov

Responsible for investigating complaints covered by regulations set forth in the Americans with Disabilities Act regarding the transportation of individuals with disabilities. Call the ADA Assistance Line, (888) 446-4511, to request a complaint form or to obtain a copy of the Americans with Disabilities Act regulations that apply to the Department of Transportation.

OFFICE OF CIVIL RIGHTS
U.S. Department of Education
300 C Street, SW
Washington, DC 20202
(800) 421-3481   (877) 521-2172 (TTY)
(202) 205-5413   FAX (202) 205-9862
www.ed.gov/offices/OCR

Responsible for enforcing laws and regulations designed to protect the rights of individuals in educational institutions that receive federal financial assistance. Individuals who feel their rights have been violated may file a complaint with one of the ten regional offices located throughout the country.

OFFICE OF FAIR HOUSING AND EQUAL OPPORTUNITY
U.S. Department of Housing and Urban Development (HUD)
451 7th Street, SW, Room 5204
Washington DC 20140
(800) 669-9777   (800) 927-9275 (TTY)
(202) 927-9275 (TTY)   www.hud.gov/fheo.html

This agency enforces the Fair Housing Act and will inform callers how to file a complaint with one of the ten regional HUD offices. Information about the Fair Housing Act and a complaint form are available on the web site.

OFFICE OF FEDERAL CONTRACT COMPLIANCE PROGRAMS (OFCCP)
U.S. Department of Labor, Employment Standards Administration
200 Constitution Avenue, NW, Room C-3325
Washington, DC 20210
(888) 378-3227   (202) 219-9475
FAX (202) 219-6195
www.dol.gov/dol/esa/ofccp/index.htm

Reviews contractors' affirmative action plans; provides technical assistance to contractors; investigates complaints; and resolves issues between contractors and employees. Ten regional offices throughout the country serve as liaisons with the national office and with district offices under their jurisdiction.

OFFICE OF GENERAL COUNSEL
U.S. Department of Transportation
400 7th Street, SW
Washington, DC 20590
(202) 366-9306   (202) 755-7687 (TTY)
FAX (202) 366-9313   www.dot.gov

Responsible for providing information and interpretation of the regulations for transportation of individuals with disabilities required by the Rehabilitation Act and the Americans with Disabilities Act. Regulations available in standard print or on audio-cassette. FREE

RURAL HOUSING SERVICE NATIONAL OFFICE
U.S. Department of Agriculture
Room 5037, South Building
14th Street and Independence Avenue, SW
Washington, DC 20250
(202) 720-4323   www.rurdev.usda.gov/rhs

Provides home ownership, renovation, and repair programs for individuals with disabilities who live in rural areas.

SOCIAL SECURITY ADMINISTRATION (SSA)
6401 Security Boulevard
Baltimore, MD 21235
(800) 772-1213   (800) 325-0778 (TTY)
www.ssa.gov

To apply for Social Security benefits based on disability, phone the number above to set up an appointment with a Social Security representative, or visit the local Social Security office. FREE interpreter services for many languages are available. Also offers FREE "e-News;" subscribe on line.

THOMAS
Library of Congress
thomas.loc.gov

This online service provides a database of recent laws and pending legislation, information about the committees of Congress, and the text of the "Congressional Record." Searches may be done by topic or public law number. Since government programs often change when they are re-authorized, this database is a good resource for the status of pending legislation.

U.S. DEPARTMENT OF HOUSING AND URBAN DEVELOPMENT (HUD)
451 7th Street, SW, Room 5240
Washington, DC 20410
(202) 708-1112   (202) 708-1455 (TTY)
www.hud.gov (HUD Section 504 One-Stop Web Site)
HUD Discrimination Hotline: (800) 669-9777; (800) 927-9275 (TTY)

Operates programs to make housing accessible, including loans for developers of independent living and group homes and loan and mortgage insurance for rehabilitation of single or multifamily units. Individuals who feel their rights have been violated may file a complaint with one of the ten regional offices located throughout the country.

PUBLICATIONS AND TAPES

THE ABA LEGAL GUIDE FOR OLDER AMERICANS
Commission on Legal Problems of the Elderly
American Bar Association
740 15th Street, NW, 9th Floor
Washington, DC 20005
(202) 662-8690   FAX (202) 662-8698
www.abanet.org/elderly

This manual provides information on subjects such as housing, health care, insurance, retirement, pensions, rights of persons with disabilities, and legal issues. $13.00

AMERICANS WITH DISABILITIES ACT: QUESTIONS AND ANSWERS
Equal Employment Opportunity Commission (EEOC)
Publications Distribution Center
PO Box 12549
Cincinnati, OH 45212-0549
(800) 669-3362   (800) 800-3302 (TTY)
FAX (513) 489-8692   www.eeoc.gov

This booklet's question and answer format provides explanations of the ADA's effects on employment, state and local governments, and public accommodations. Available in standard print, alternate formats, automated fax system, and on the web site. FREE. Also available at www.pueblo.gsa.gov. Click on "Federal Programs."

DIRECTORY OF LEGAL AID AND DEFENDER OFFICES
National Legal Aid and Defender Association
1625 K Street, NW, 8th Floor
Washington, DC 20006
(202) 452-0620   FAX (202) 872-1031
www.nlads.org

A directory of legal aid offices throughout the U.S. Includes chapters on disability protection/advocacy, health law, and senior citizens. Updated biennially. $70.00

FEDERAL BENEFITS FOR VETERANS AND DEPENDENTS
Federal Consumer Information Center
PO Box 100
Pueblo, CO 81002
(888) 878-3256   www.pueblo.gsa.gov

This booklet describes the benefits available under federal laws. $5.00. Also available on the web site. Click on "Federal Programs."

FEDERAL REGISTER
New Orders, Superintendent of Documents
PO Box 371954
Pittsburgh, PA 15250-7954
(866) 512-1800   (202) 512-1530
FAX (202) 512-2250
www.access.gpo.gov/su_docs/aces/aces140.html

A federal publication printed every weekday with notices of all regulations and legal notices issued by federal agencies. Domestic subscriptions, $764.00 annually for second class mailing of paper format; $264.00 annually for microfiche. Access to the Federal Register is available through the Internet at the address listed above. FREE

A GUIDE TO DISABILITY RIGHTS LAWS
Federal Consumer Information Center
PO Box 100
Pueblo, CO 81002
(888) 878-3256   www.pueblo.gsa.gov

This brochure summarizes federal laws that are applicable to individuals with disabilities and lists the agencies that enforce them. FREE. Also available on the web site.

A GUIDE TO LEGAL RIGHTS FOR PEOPLE WITH DISABILITIES
by Marc D. Stolman
Demos Medical Publishing
386 Park Avenue South, Suite 201
New York, NY 10016
(800) 532-8663   (212) 683-0072
www.demosmedpub.com

This book discusses civil rights, insurance, benefits, and legal issues faced by individuals with disabilities. $24.95. Orders made on the Demos web site receive a 15% discount.

GUIDE TO USING THE FAMILY AND MEDICAL LEAVE ACT: QUESTIONS AND ANSWERS
National Partnership for Women and Families
1875 Connecticut Avenue, NW, Suite 710
Washington, DC 20009
(202) 986-2600   FAX (202) 986-2539
www.nationalpartnership.org

This booklet answers the most frequently asked questions about the law. Available in English and Spanish. FREE. Also available on the web site.

INSURANCE SOLUTIONS--PLAN WELL, LIVE BETTER: A WORKBOOK FOR PEOPLE WITH CHRONIC ILLNESSES OR DISABILITIES
by Laura D. Cooper
Demos Medical Publishing
386 Park Avenue South, Suite 201
New York, NY 10016
(800) 532-8663   (212) 683-0072
FAX (212) 683-0118   www.demosmedpub.com

This book enables readers to find and evaluate insurance options. Includes checklists, worksheets, and exercises. $24.95. Orders made on the Demos web site receive a 15% discount.

KNOW YOUR RIGHTS
National Technical Information Service (NTIS)
5285 Port Royal Road
Springfield, VA 22161
(800) 553-6847   (703) 605-4600
FAX (703) 605-6900   www.ntis.gov

This videotape explains the legal rights of residents in nursing homes, using actual examples. Available in English and Spanish. 9 minutes. $50.00

LAWS ENFORCED BY THE U.S. EQUAL EMPLOYMENT OPPORTUNITY COMMISSION
Equal Employment Opportunity Commission (EEOC)
Publications Distribution Center
PO Box 12549
Cincinnati, OH 45212-0549
(800) 669-3362   (800) 800-3302 (TTY)
FAX (513) 489-8692   www.eeoc.gov

Included in this booklet are Title VII of the Civil Rights Act of 1964, Equal Pay Act, Age Discrimination in Employment Act, Rehabilitation Act of 1973, Title I of the Americans with Disabilities Act, and the Civil Rights Act of 1991. FREE

MEDICARE & YOU
Centers for Medicare and Medicaid Services (CMS)
formerly Health Care Financing Administration (HCFA)
7500 Security Boulevard
Baltimore, MD 21244
(800) 633-4227   (877) 486-2048
(410) 786-3000   cms.hhs.gov
www.medicare.gov

This booklet provides basic information about Medicare, including eligibility, enrollment, coverage, and options. Available in English and Spanish in standard print and alternate formats. FREE. Also available on the web site.

MEETING THE NEEDS OF EMPLOYEES WITH DISABILITIES
Resources for Rehabilitation
22 Bonad Road
Winchester, MA 01890
(781) 368-9094   FAX (781) 368-9096
www.rfr.org

This book provides information to help people with disabilities retain or obtain employment. Chapters on vision, mobility, and hearing and speech impairments include information on organizations, products, and services. $44.95. See order form on last page of this book.

RETIREMENT BENEFITS
SOCIAL SECURITY DISABILITY PROGRAMS CAN HELP
SOCIAL SECURITY: WHAT YOU NEED TO KNOW WHEN YOU GET
DISABILITY BENEFITS
WORKING WHILE DISABLED... HOW WE CAN HELP
Social Security Administration
(800) 772-1213   (800) 325-0778 (TTY)
www.ssa.gov

These booklets provide basic information about Social Security programs for individuals with disabilities. The Social Security Administration distributes many other titles, including many that are available in alternate formats and in Spanish. Publications are available on the web site and at local Social Security offices. FREE

SOCIAL SECURITY, MEDICARE, AND PENSIONS:
THE SOURCEBOOK FOR OLDER AMERICANS
by Joseph Matthews and Dorothy Matthews Berman
Nolo Press
950 Parker Street
Berkeley, CA 94710
(800) 992-6656   (510) 549-1976
FAX (800) 645-0895   www.nolo.com

This book provides information on Social Security, Medicare and Medicaid, Supplemental Security Income, veterans' benefits, and civil service benefits. It also discusses a variety of Internet sites related to these topics. $29.95

A SUMMARY OF DEPARTMENT OF VETERANS AFFAIRS BENEFITS
(800) 827-1000   www.va.gov

This booklet is available from any VA regional office. FREE

Chapter 3
MAKING EVERYDAY LIVING SAFER AND EASIER

The increase in the number of elders and others with disabilities has generated an expanding marketplace of programs and products that facilitate independent living. Consideration of housing alternatives and utilization of assistive devices go a long way to help elders feel safe and comfortable in their own homes. This chapter provides information about fall prevention, housing options, and products that enable elders to continue living in the community; engage in their everyday activities, including work; and travel in comfort.

The overwhelming majority of elders live in the community and nearly one-third live alone (U.S. Department of Health and Human Services: 1991). It is very important that they have the information that enables them to live comfortably and without fear, no matter what their living arrangements. Information about environmental adaptations and assistive devices related to specific disabilities is presented in earlier chapters which focus on these disabilities (e.g., hearing loss, vision loss, etc.).

FALLS AND SAFETY

It has been estimated that a third of noninstitutionalized individuals age 65 or over fall each year; among elders in long term care facilities, the proportion is higher. In most cases, falls do not cause serious injuries, although more than 215,000 falls each year result in hip fractures (National Institute on Aging: 1991). Hip fractures, in turn, may lead to other health problems and a consequent loss of independence. Stevens and her colleagues (1999) report that 50% of elders who fracture a hip do not return to their former functional level.

Risk factors for falls include the use of sedatives, cognitive impairment, alcohol consumption, and posture and gait problems. In addition, osteoporosis, Parkinson's disease, stroke, and visual impairment are predisposing factors for falls. Environmental hazards are also the source of a large proportion of falls. Many elders have multiple disabilities that are risk factors for falls, and often the exact cause (or causes) of a given fall is unknown.

Tinetti and her colleagues (1988) found that nearly one-third (32%) of individuals 75 years or older living in the community fell at least once during their one year study. Of those who fell, one-quarter (24%) sustained serious injuries.

Several investigators have suggested that the fear of falling itself results in the self-imposed limitation of activity by many elders (Duthie: 1989; Tinetti et al.: 1988). One study (Walker and Howland: 1991) found that fear of falling resulted in the curtailment of activities by 41% of the respondents.

Ironically, the fear of falling may actually result in additional falls, because inactivity may cause weakness and hinder joint mobility (Sattin: 1992; Walker and Howland: 1991). Research has confirmed that exercise may play a protective role in preventing fractures among elders (National Institute on Aging: 1991; Sorock et al.: 1988). Health care professionals, especially physical therapists, can help develop walking and exercise programs that build muscle strength and enable elders to continue to be active.

The American Geriatrics Society (2001) identified six major risk factors for falls: muscle weakness, a history of falls, gait deficits, balance deficits, use of an assistive device, and visual deficit. The Society released clinical guidelines to assess and reduce these risk factors and published a consumer guide (see "PUBLICATIONS AND TAPES" below).

Since most falls in the older population occur in the home, environmental adaptations may reduce the occurrence of falls and provide reassurance to elders who have fallen in the past and fear falling again. There are many obvious ways of making the home safer and preventing falls; these include using nonskid rugs, providing good lighting and reducing glare, installing grab bars in tubs and next to toilets, using chairs in the shower, and eliminating elevated thresholds. Level, nonskid floors, uncluttered aisles, and handrails along stairs may also help to prevent falls. The use of canes and other mobility aids may assist elders who have trouble walking and bolster their confidence as well.

Personal response systems for emergencies may reduce the fear of falling, fostering self-confidence in elders with disabilities and enabling family members or other caregivers to feel comfortable when leaving the home. If an individual falls or experiences symptoms of a medical emergency, he or she activates the system, usually by pushing a device that is worn around the neck or kept nearby, that alerts a designated response network. Purchase and installation of equipment may be reimbursable by third-party payment, although the individual is usually responsible for monthly service fees.

Public health officials, recognizing that falls among elders pose a serious health problem, have suggested that prevention programs be implemented on a widespread basis. Using the risk factors associated with falling to determine the target population, occupational therapists, architects, and others trained in environmental adaptations could conduct environmental assessments of the home environments of elders as well as places that they frequent, such as senior centers and churches. Checklists of home safety items are available from a number of organizations to facilitate this undertaking (See "PUBLICATIONS AND TAPES" section below).

REFERENCES

American Geriatrics Society
2001 "Guideline for the Prevention of Falls in Older Persons" JOURNAL OF THE AMERICAN GERIATRICS SOCIETY 48:5(May):664-672

Duthie, Edmund H.
1989 "Falls" MEDICAL CLINICS OF NORTH AMERICA
73(November):6:1321-1336
National Institute on Aging
1991 PHYSICAL FRAILTY Department of Health and Human
Services, NIH Publication 91-397
Sattin, Richard W.
1992 "Falls among Older Persons: A Public Health Perspective"
ANNUAL REVIEW OF PUBLIC HEALTH 13:489-508
Sorock, Gary S. et al.
1988 "Physical Activity and Fracture Risk in a Free-Living Elderly
Cohort" JOURNAL OF GERONTOLOGY MEDICAL
SCIENCES 43:5:M134-139
Stevens, J.A. et al.
1999 "Surveillance for Injuries and Violence in Older Adults"
CDC SURVEILLANCE SUMMARIES 48:SS-8(December
17):27-50
Tinetti, Mary E., Mark Speechley, and Sandra F. Ginter
1988 "Risk Factors for Falls among Elderly Persons Living in the
Community" NEW ENGLAND JOURNAL OF MEDICINE
349:26:1701-1707
Walker, J. Elizabeth and Jonathan Howland
1991 "Falls and Fear of Falling among Elderly Persons Living in
the Community: Occupational Therapy Interventions"
AMERICAN JOURNAL OF OCCUPATIONAL THERAPY
45:2(February):119-122
U.S. Department of Health and Human Services
1991 AGING IN AMERICA TRENDS AND PROJECTIONS DHHS
Publication No. (FCoA) 91-28001

ORGANIZATIONS

AMERICAN ACADEMY OF ORTHOPAEDIC SURGEONS
6300 North River Road
Rosemont, IL 60018
(800) 346-2267   (847) 823-7186
FAX (847) 823-8125   orthoinfo.aaos.org

A professional organization for orthopaedic surgeons and allied health professionals. Web site offers links such as "Prevent Falls" and "Find a Surgeon." Fact sheets available online include "Getting Up From a Fall," "Don't Let a Fall Be Your Last Trip," and "Home Safety Checklist." A quarterly e-mail newsletter, "Your Orthopaedic Connection," is available upon request.

MEDLINEPLUS: EXERCISE FOR SENIORS
www.nlm.nih.gov/medlineplus/exerciseforseniors.html

This web site provides links to sites for information about exercise for seniors, including disease management, prevention/screening, organizations, and specific conditions/aspects. Includes an interactive tutorial on exercising for a healthy heart. Provides links to MEDLINE research articles and related MEDLINEplus pages.

MEDLINEPLUS: FALLS
www.nlm.nih.gov/medlineplus/falls.html

This web site provides links to sites for general information about falls, prevention and screening, specific conditions/aspects, organizations, and statistics. Provides links to MEDLINE research articles and related MEDLINEplus pages.

NATIONAL ALLIANCE TO PREVENT FALLS AS WE AGE
National Safety Council
1121 Spring Lake Drive
Itasca, IL 60143
(630) 285-1121   www.nsc.org

The members of the Alliance work to educate the public about fall prevention, home modification, and physical activity to promote balance and strength.

NIH SENIOR HEALTH
nihseniorhealth.gov

This web site provides information on topics such as exercise for older adults. Includes video demonstrations of strength, balance, stretching, and endurance exercises that may be watched online.

PUBLICATIONS AND TAPES

CHECK FOR SAFETY: A HOME FALL PREVENTION CHECKLIST FOR OLDER ADULTS
National Center for Injury Prevention and Control
4770 Buford Highway, NE, Mailstop K65
Atlanta, GA 30341-3724
(770) 488-1506   www.cdc.gov/ncipc

This checklist enables individuals to identify and remedy hazards in areas such as floors, stairs and steps, kitchen, bedrooms, and bathrooms. Available in English and Spanish. LARGE PRINT. FREE

EXERCISE: A GUIDE FROM THE NATIONAL INSTITUTE ON AGING
National Institute on Aging Information Center
PO Box 8057
Gaithersburg, MD 20898-8057
(800) 222-2225   www.nia.nih.gov

This videotape demonstrates stretching, balance, and strength-training exercises. 48 minutes. $7.00. Includes 80 page companion booklet.

FALL PREVENTION
Osteoporosis and Related Bone Diseases National Resource Center (ORBD)
1150 17th Street, Suite 500
Washington, DC 20036-4603
(800) 624-2663   (202) 223-0344
(202) 466-4315 (TTY)   FAX (202) 223-2237
www.osteo.org

This fact sheet provides indoor and outdoor safety tips and discusses adaptations to prevent falls. FREE

HOME SAFETY CHECKLIST FOR OLDER CONSUMERS
U.S. Consumer Product Safety Commission
Washington, DC 20207
(800) 638-2772   www.cpsc.gov

Provides information on simple, inexpensive repairs and safety recommendations. Available in English and Spanish. FREE. Also available on the web site.

PATIENT'S GUIDE TO PREVENTING FALLS
American Geriatrics Society
350 Fifth Avenue, Suite 801
New York, NY 10118
(212) 308-1414   FAX (212) 832-8646
www.americangeriatrics.org

This leaflet provides information on simple interventions that may reduce the risk of falls. Includes a medication chart. FREE. Also available on the web site.

PREVENTING FALLS
Terra Nova Films, Inc.
9848 South Winchester Avenue
Chicago, IL 60643
(800) 779-8491   (773) 881-8491
www.terranova.org

This videotape reviews hazardous situations that can lead to falls. Includes printed checklists of hazards and tips to assess risks. 17 minutes. $119.00

PREVENTING FALLS: A DEFENSIVE APPROACH
by J. Thomas Hutton
Prometheus Books
59 John Glenn Drive
Amherst, NY 14228
(800) 421-0351   FAX (716) 691-0137
www.prometheusbooks.com

This book describes the Defensive Falls School, a program designed to help individuals with Parkinson's disease and others who are at risk for falls. Discusses topics such as vision, balance, gait, posture, and freezing; provides home safety assessments and transfer techniques; and suggests environmental changes. $19.00. A videotape that demonstrates preventive strategies is also available. 60 minutes. $22.00

SAFE LIVING WITH PEACE OF MIND
A/V Health Services
PO Box 20271
Roanoke, VA 24018-0028
(540) 725-9288 (Voice and FAX)
www.avhealthservices.com

This videotape enables individuals to assess home safety. Demonstrates simple modifications, adaptive equipment, and safety techniques. 25 minutes. $45.00

HOUSING

Elders who find it increasingly difficult to maintain their own homes due to physical or economic constraints have a number of housing options available to them. Many elders are ineligible for governmental housing subsidy programs because they own their homes. Real estate taxes and home repair, maintenance and adaptation costs consume a large percentage of their annual income. To ameliorate these situations, the Department of Housing and Urban Development (HUD) offers several housing assistance programs.

HOME EQUITY CONVERSION MORTGAGES, sometimes called reverse mortgages, are insured by HUD in the event that the lender defaults and allow elders to convert the equity in their homes into cash that will enable them to meet housing expenses. The reverse mortgage does not have to be repaid until the mortgagee moves or dies. Homeowners must be age 62 or older, occupy their own home as a principal residence, and own the home free and clear or nearly so. Reverse mortgage payment options include "tenure," monthly payments to homeowners as long as they use their homes as principal residences; "term," which provides monthly payments for a specified period; and "line-of-credit," which allows homeowners to draw on their equity up to a maximum amount.

PUBLIC HOUSING is a major housing resource for elders with low income. SECTION 8 Certificates and Vouchers provide federal subsidies to income-eligible households to help defray housing costs in the private rental market. Section 8 subsidies may also be used in group shared residences and for homeownership. Local public housing authorities administer the program. Section 803 of the National Affordable Housing Act of 1990, HOPE for Elderly Independence, combines tenant-based rental housing certificates and rental vouchers with supportive services to enable frail elders who have not been receiving any form of housing assistance to continue living in the community. (For additional information on laws pertaining to housing, see Chapter 2, "Laws that Affect Elders with Disabilities.")

Other housing options for elders include ASSISTED LIVING FACILITIES, such as board and care homes, adult care homes, and residential care facilities; these facilities provide personal assistance with medications and other daily activities, as needed. CONTINUING CARE RETIREMENT COMMUNITIES provide housing choices ranging from independent apartment living with services such as congregate meals and activities to 24-hour nursing care. ACCESSORY HOUSING, independent housing units built on to single family homes or erected on the property of a single family home, is another option for elders who wish to live independently but need supportive services.

NATURALLY OCCURRING RETIREMENT COMMUNITIES represent a recent trend of elders to move into apartment buildings that are convenient to public transportation, shopping, and other necessary services. Although not officially recognized as housing for elders, these buildings house a high proportion of elders. As a result, property managers are beginning to employ social workers and community agencies to provide the services needed by their tenants.

SHARED HOUSING is another option that may enable elders to stay in their own homes or to move into someone else's home. Elders who live alone may find it financially tenable to stay in their homes if another person moves in to share the costs. When other elders move in, the tasks of maintaining a home may also become more manageable. In some instances, elders share their homes with younger individuals, often students who need a low cost place to live and in return carry out some of the chores that the elders are unable to do. Group residences, where elders share meals and facilities, are another option.

Many state offices on aging publish directories of assisted living facilities, retirement communities, subsidized housing, and shared housing. These directories often include checklists that individuals may use in evaluating these facilities.

Elders who wish to remain in their own homes may find that environmental adaptations enable them to do so. For example, the installation of ramps, elevators, and special lifts to climb the stairs may be sufficient for elders with mobility impairments. Lowered kitchen counters and appliances facilitate cooking for individuals who use wheelchairs. Other adaptive design features include accessible routes, light switches, electrical outlets, and thermostats; bathrooms with walls sturdy enough to install grab bars; and kitchens and bathrooms with sufficient space to maneuver wheelchairs.

Many architects now specialize in designing buildings and dwelling units that meet the needs of people with disabilities. The state office on disability, the architectural access board, or the local or state professional society of architects should be able to provide a list of qualified architects.

ORGANIZATIONS

ABLEDATA
8630 Fenton Street, Suite 930
Silver Spring, MD 20910
(800) 227-0216   www.abledata.com

This federally funded center responds to telephone, mail, and e-mail inquiries about disabilities, assistive products, and support services. Most publications may be downloaded from the web site.

AMERICAN ASSOCIATION OF HOMES AND SERVICES FOR THE AGED (AAHSA)
2519 Connecticut Avenue, NW
Washington, DC 20008
(800) 675-9253   (202) 783-2242
FAX (202) 783-2255   www.aahsa.org

The AAHSA is a national association of nonprofit organizations that provide housing and health care to elders. The Continuing Care Accreditation Commission, part of the AAHSA, accredits continuing care retirement communities throughout the country. The web site offers "Consumer Tips" on subjects such as "Choosing an Assisted Living Facility" and "Finding the Right Nursing Home."

ARCHITECTURAL AND TRANSPORTATION BARRIERS COMPLIANCE BOARD (ATBCB)
1331 F Street, NW, Suite 1000
Washington, DC 20004-1111
(800) 872-2253   (800) 993-2822 (TTY)
(202) 272-0080   (202) 272-0082 (TTY)
FAX (202) 272-0081   www.access-board.gov

A federal agency charged with developing standards for accessibility in federal facilities, public accommodations, and transportation facilities as required by the Americans with Disabilities Act and other federal laws. Provides technical assistance, sponsors research, and distributes publications. Publishes a quarterly newsletter, "Access America." All publications available in standard print, alternate formats, and on the web site; FREE.

ASSISTED LIVING FEDERATION OF AMERICA (ALFA)
11200 Waples Mill Road, Suite 150
Fairfax, VA 22030
(800) 258-7030   (703) 691-8100
FAX (703) 691-8106   www.alfa.org

Trade association of assisted living facilities. State by state listing of facilities and checklist for evaluating facilities available on request. FREE. Also available on web site.

CENTER FOR UNIVERSAL DESIGN
North Carolina State University
219 Oberlin Road
Raleigh, NC 27695
(800) 647-6777   (919) 515-3082 (V/TTY)
FAX (919) 515-3023   www.design.ncsu.edu/cud

A federally funded research and training center that works toward improving housing and product design for people with disabilities. Provides technical assistance, training, and publications. Some publications are available on the web site.

ELDERNET
1330 Beacon Street, Suite 268
Brookline, MA 02446
(617) 244-1774   www.eldernet.com

Developed by an attorney who specializes in issues that affect elders, this web site provides information and links related to health, housing, finances, laws, and retirement.

FANNIE MAE
(800) 732-6643   www.fanniemae.com

This private company offers mortgage products designed to help individuals with disabilities attain home ownership. Publishes "A Home of Your Own Guide," for housing educators and counselors who work with individuals with disabilities; available through the Fannie Mae Distribution Center, (800) 471-5554. FREE. Also available on the web site.

GE ANSWER CENTER
Louisville, KY 40222
(800) 626-2000   (800) 833-4322 (TTY)

This consumer information center provides assistance to individuals with disabilities as well as to the general public. Appliance controls marked with braille or raised dots are available for individuals who are blind or visually impaired, FREE. Two brochures, "Real Life Design" (available in standard print and alternate formats) and "Basic Kitchen Planning for the Physically Handicapped," are FREE. The center is open 24 hours a day, seven days a week.

MEDLINEPLUS: ASSISTED LIVING
www.nlm.nih.gov/medlineplus/assistedliving.html

This web site provides links to sites for general information about assisted living. Includes information about specific conditions and aspects, law and policy, directories, and organizations. Some information is available in Spanish. Provides links to MEDLINE research articles and related MEDLINEplus pages.

NATIONAL ASSOCIATION OF HOME BUILDERS (NAHB)
National Research Center, Economics and Policy Analysis
Division
400 Prince George's Boulevard
Upper Marlboro, MD 20772
(301) 249-4000   FAX (301) 430-6180
www.nahbrc.org

The research section of the home building industry trade
organization produces publications and provides training on
housing and special needs.

NATIONAL COUNCIL OF STATE HOUSING AGENCIES (NCSHA)
444 North Capitol Street, NW, Suite 438
Washington, DC 20001
(202) 624-7710   FAX (202) 624-5899
www.ncsha.org

Membership organization of state housing agencies. Web site
offers a "State Housing Finance Agency Directory" that lists
assistance available for home modifications and home ownership
programs.

NATIONAL HOME OF YOUR OWN ALLIANCE
Center for Housing and New Community Economics
Institute on Disability
University of New Hampshire
7 Leavitt Lane, Suite 101
Durham, NH 03824
(800) 220-8770   alliance.unh.edu

The web site provides extensive information about housing for individuals with disabilities, including the Section 8 Homeownership Rule; "A Home of Your Own Guide" for prospective home

owners; and information about state housing coalitions, funding sources, and other resources.

NATIONAL SHARED HOUSING RESOURCE CENTER (NSHRC)
5342 Tilly Mill Road
Dunwoody, GA 30338
www.nationalsharedhousing.org

Directs elders to homesharing programs in their area and provides technical assistance in program development. Publishes the "Shared Housing Directory," a state-by-state listing; $20.00; also available on the web site. Membership, individuals, $20.00; professionals, $50.00; includes quarterly newsletter, "Consumer's Guide to Home Sharing."

RETIREMENT LIVING INFORMATION CENTER
www.retirementliving.com

This web site provides information about retirement communities and other senior housing as well as links to state aging agencies, vendors of special products, and other resources.

RURAL HOUSING SERVICE NATIONAL OFFICE
U.S. Department of Agriculture
Room 5037, South Building
14th Street and Independence Avenue, SW
Washington, DC 20250
(202) 720-4323   www.rurdev.usda.gov/rhs

Provides home ownership, renovation, and repair programs for individuals with disabilities who live in rural areas.

PUBLICATIONS AND TAPES

ADAPTING THE HOME FOR THE PHYSICALLY CHALLENGED
A/V Health Services
PO Box 20271
Roanoke, VA 24018-0028
(540) 725-9288 (Voice and FAX)
www.avhealthservices.com

This videotape will assist individuals who use wheelchairs or walkers modify their homes. Ramp construction and modifications for every room are explained. 30 minutes. $70.00

A CONSUMER'S GUIDE TO HOME ADAPTATION
Adaptive Environments Center
374 Congress Street, Suite 301
Boston, MA 02210
(617) 695-1225 (V/TTY)   FAX (617) 482-8099
www.adaptenvironments.org

This workbook enables people with disabilities to plan the modifications necessary to adapt their homes. Describes how to widen doorways, lower countertops, etc. $12.00

THE CONTINUING CARE RETIREMENT COMMUNITY:
A GUIDEBOOK FOR CONSUMERS
American Association of Homes and Services for the Aged
PO Box 1616
1650 Blue Grass Lakes Highway
Alpharetta, GA 30009
(800) 675-9253   www.aahsa.org

This book describes continuing care retirement community contracts and provides a checklist and financial worksheet. $10.45

DESIGNS FOR INDEPENDENT LIVING
THE LESS CHALLENGING HOME
Appliance Information Service
Whirlpool Corporation
Benton Harbor, MI 49022
(800) 253-1301   (800) 334-6889 (TTY)
www.whirlpool.com

The first brochure provides information on adaptations for the home environment and major appliances. FREE. The second booklet provides suggestions for incorporating accessible design when building or remodeling kitchens and bathrooms. Describes building materials and appliances and includes charts indicating appliance features that are helpful to users with disabilities. FREE

DIRECTORY OF ACCESSIBLE BUILDING PRODUCTS
National Association of Home Builders (NAHB)
National Research Center, Economics and Policy Analysis Division
400 Prince George's Boulevard
Upper Marlboro, MD 20772
(301) 249-4000   FAX (301) 430-6180
www.nahbrc.org

This directory describes and illustrates products available for use by individuals with disabilities. $5.00

EASY THINGS TO MAKE--TO MAKE THINGS EASY: SIMPLE DO-IT-YOURSELF HOME MODIFICATIONS FOR OLDER PEOPLE AND OTHERS WITH PHYSICAL DISABILITIES by Doreen Greenstein
Brookline Books
PO Box 1047
Cambridge, MA 02238-1047
(800) 666-2665   (617) 868-0360
FAX (617) 868-1772   www.brooklinebooks.com

This book describes low-cost home modifications and suggests adaptations for everyday activities. LARGE PRINT. $15.95

HOME MADE MONEY: A CONSUMER'S GUIDE TO REVERSE MORTGAGES
AARP
formerly American Association of Retired Persons
601 E Street, NW
Washington DC 20049
(800) 424-3410   www.aarp.org

This booklet discusses this option and compares the types of loans and borrower decisions. FREE. Also available on the web site.

HOMESHARING: MATCHING FOR INDEPENDENCE
National Shared Housing Resource Center
5342 Tilly Mill Road
Dunwoody, GA 30338
www.nationalsharedhousing.org

A guide for developing match-up programs for elders who want to share housing. Professional members, $30.00; nonmembers, $35.00.

HOW TO BUILD RAMPS FOR HOME ACCESSIBILITY
Metropolitan Center for Independent Living
1600 University Avenue West, Suite 16
St. Paul, MN 55104-3825
(651) 603-2029   www.wheelchairramp.org

The manual and videotape provide step-by-step instruction in building modular ramps and steps. Manual, $15.00. May also be downloaded from web site. Videotape, $20.00.

IMPROVING THE QUALITY OF LONG-TERM CARE
by Gooloo S. Wunderlich and Peter O. Kohler (eds.)
National Academy Press
2101 Constitution Avenue, NW
Lockbox 285
Washington, DC 20055
(888) 624-8373   (202) 334-3313
FAX (202) 334-2451   www.nap.edu

The report of the Committee on Improving Quality in Long-Term Care, this book looks at the current status of care and quality of life in nursing homes and other residential care communities as well as health agencies. It identifies problems and makes recommendations for government agencies. $47.95. A 20% discount is offered for purchases made on the web site. May be read on the web site, FREE.

LINKING HOUSING AND HEALTH SERVICES FOR OLDER PERSONS
Milbank Memorial Fund
645 Madison Avenue
New York, NY 10022
(212) 355-8400

This report describes programs which integrate health care and supportive services into housing for elders to promote independence. FREE

REMOVING BARRIERS TO HEALTH CARE: A GUIDE FOR HEALTH PROFESSIONALS
Center for Universal Design
North Carolina State University
219 Oberlin Road
Raleigh, NC 27695
(800) 647-6777   (919) 515-3082 (V/TTY)
FAX (919) 515-3023   www.design.ncsu.edu/cud

This booklet provides guidelines for access to health care facilities. Reviews the design standards of the Americans with Disabilities Act and suggests methods for courteous interactions with individuals with disabilities. FREE

RETROFITTING HOMES FOR A LIFETIME
National Association of Home Builders (NAHB)
National Research Center, Economics and Policy Analysis Division
400 Prince George's Boulevard
Upper Marlboro, MD 20772-8731
(301) 249-4000   FAX (301) 430-6180
www.nahbrc.org

This publication enables remodelers and homeowners to assess needed modifications; provides an accessibility checklist; suggests financing alternatives; and makes recommendations for working with builders. $15.00

SHARED HOUSING FOR THE ELDERLY
by Dale Jaffe (ed.)
Greenwood Publishing Group
88 Post Road West
Westport, CT 06881
(800) 225-5800   (203) 226-3571
FAX (203) 222-1502   www.greenwood.com

A series of articles about the advantages and problems of shared
housing programs. $69.95

RECREATION AND TRAVEL

Travel and recreation opportunities for elders with disabilities have expanded greatly in recent years. Some elders with disabilities need assistance in order to continue with their favorite hobbies or recreational pastimes. Others may develop an interest in a new hobby or sport as a means of socializing with organized groups or individuals. Staff at the agencies that serve elders can make referrals to organizations and groups that offer programs such as adult education courses and adapted exercise programs.

Many state tourism offices will provide information about accessible attractions for prospective visitors with disabilities, as will the tourist office of many foreign countries. Auto clubs both here and abroad are also good sources for such information.

The Americans with Disabilities Act (ADA) of 1990 mandates accessibility to recreation facilities and athletic programs, from aerobic training classes and local parks to football stadiums and other venues. Advances in technology have led to the development of racing wheelchairs, special hand and foot prostheses, and adapted ski equipment such as sit-skis. All-terrain vehicles (ATVs), adapted with lifts, hand controls, or safety harnesses, enable individuals with mobility impairments to participate in many outdoor recreation activities.

The ADA also requires that fixed route buses and rail transportation be accessible to individuals with disabilities. However, deadlines for implementation of the ADA's regulations vary from six to seven years for private intercity transit to as long as 20 years for Amtrak and commuter rail stations. Many communities offer special transportation services for elders and for individuals with disabilities for a nominal fee. These services enable elders to shop on their own, participate in recreational activities, visit friends and relatives, and go to the offices of health care providers.

The Federal Aviation Administration requires each airline to submit a company-wide policy for travelers with disabilities.

Passengers may call ahead to request early boarding, special seating, or meals which meet dietary restrictions. Airport facilities are designed to offer accessible restrooms, elevators, electric carts or wheelchairs, and first aid stations. The Air Carrier Access Act of 1986 (ACAA) contains regulations that cover the needs of travelers with disabilities, such as access to commuter planes, accessible lavatories, wheelchair storage, and sensitivity training for all airline personnel. Contact the airlines to obtain a written statement of the special services they provide. Individuals who believe that their rights have been denied may file a complaint within 45 days of the incident with the Department of Transportation, Office of Consumer Affairs, C-75 Room 4107, Washington, DC 20590, (202) 366-2220; www.dot.gov/airconsumer

Amtrak offers a 15% discount on regular one-way coach travel and accessible sleeping accommodations for adults with disabilities. Passengers must present proof of disability, such as a certificate of legal blindness or a letter from a physician specifying the nature of the disability. The discount also applies to a companion fare. Greyhound allows passengers with disabilities requiring assistance with personal hygiene, eating, medications, or while the bus is in motion to request a FREE ticket for a companion (certain restrictions apply). There is no charge for service dogs for individuals who are visually impaired, blind, or deaf.

Travel agencies that plan special trips for people with disabilities are available throughout the country. Many major hotel chains, airlines, and car rental companies provide special assistance to people with disabilities and often have special toll-free numbers for users of text telephones. Some companies offer specially trained travel companions to people with disabilities who need an escort.

Individuals with disabilities and elders are eligible for special entrance passes to federal recreation facilities. The Golden Access Passport is a FREE lifetime pass available to any U.S. citizen or permanent resident, regardless of age, who is blind or permanently disabled. It admits the permit holder and passengers in a single, private, noncommercial vehicle to any parks, monuments, historic sites, recreation areas and wildlife refuges which usually charge entrance fees. If the permit holder does not enter by car, the Passport admits the permit holder, spouse, and children. The permit holder is also entitled to a 50% discount on charges such as camping, boat launching, and parking fees. Fees charged by private concessionaires are not discounted. Golden Access Passports are available only in person, with proof of disability, such as a certificate of legal blindness. A Golden Age Passport offers the same benefits to persons age 62 or older, with proof of age. Since the Passport is available at most federal recreation areas, it is not necessary to obtain one ahead of time.

Many Department of Veterans Affairs Medical Centers offer driver evaluation services, driving training instruction, and information services to veterans with disabilities through the Rehabilitation Medicine Service at their facilities. The AARP (American Association of Retired Persons) offers classroom refresher courses for drivers 50 years of age and over. The Internal Revenue Service allows individuals to include in medical expenses the cost of special hand controls and other special equipment installed in a car to be used by a person with a disability. Individuals may also consider as a medical expense the difference between the cost of a car designed to hold a wheelchair and the cost of the car without modification. Contact the Internal Revenue Service (see "ORGANIZATIONS" section below) to obtain Publication 502 "Medical and Dental Expenses." Major automobile manufacturers offer reimbursement for adaptive equipment installed on new vehicles. Programs for special adaptive equipment offered by automobile manufacturers are listed in the "ORGANIZATIONS" section below.

ORGANIZATIONS

ACCESS-ABLE TRAVEL SERVICE
PO Box 1796
Wheat Ridge, CO 80034
(303) 232-2979   FAX (303) 239-8486
www.access-able.com

Provides information on accommodations, access guides, entertainment, tours, and transportation. FREE monthly newsletter available by e-mail.

ACCESS OUTDOORS
www.accessoutdoors.org

This web site provides information about organizations that offer accessible outdoor recreation experiences, adaptive recreation products, and organizations that provide assistance in creating accessible programs. A service of Wilderness Inquiry.

ACHILLES TRACK CLUB
42 West 38th Street, 4th Floor
New York, NY 10018
(212) 354-0300   FAX (212) 354-3978
www.achillestrackclub.org

Promotes running as a recreational activity and competitive sport for individuals with disabilities. Chapters in many states and foreign countries. Membership is FREE. Publishes newsletter, "The Achilles Heel."

ADED - ASSOCIATION FOR DRIVER REHABILITATION SPECIALISTS
711 South Vienna Street
Ruston, LA 71270
(800) 290-2344   (318) 257-5055
FAX (318) 255-4175   www.driver-ed.org

Certifies members to conduct driver evaluation and training for individuals with disabilities.

AIR TRAVEL CONSUMER REPORT
www.dot.gov/airconsumer/disabled.htm

This web site includes information about the rights of passengers with disabilities. The rights of individuals with disabilities regarding new security regulations issued in late 2001 are described in a fact sheet at www.dot/gov/airconsumer/01-index.htm.

AMTRAK
(877) 268-7252   (800) 523-6590 (TTY)
www.amtrak.com

Provides 15% discount on most fares, including accessible sleeping accommodations, for individuals with disabilities. Also applies to companion fare. On-board services and special meals available upon request with advance notice. Request "Access Amtrak: A Guide to Amtrak Services for Travelers with Disabilities." Available in standard print and alternate formats. FREE

ARCHITECTURAL AND TRANSPORTATION BARRIERS COMPLIANCE BOARD (ATBCB)

1331 F Street, NW, Suite 1000
Washington, DC 20004

(800) 872-2253	(800) 993-2822 (TTY)
(202) 272-0080	(202) 272-0082 (TTY)
FAX (202) 272-0081	www.access-board.gov

Maintains a database on accessible transportation, including an annotated bibliography. Publishes brochures on subjects such as "Air Carrier Policies on Transport of Battery Powered Wheelchairs."

AUTO CHANNEL

(877) 275-4226   www.ican.com

Provides a step-by-step evaluation to enable consumers with disabilities to choose the vehicle that meets their needs.

AUTOMOBILITY

DaimlerChrysler Corporation
PO Box 5080
Troy, MI 48007-5080

(800) 255-9877	(800) 922-3826 (TTY)
FAX (810) 597-3501	

www.automobility.daimlerchrysler.com

Provides $750 to $1000 reimbursement (on eligible models) on the purchase of alerting devices for people who are deaf or hearing impaired and assistive equipment for vehicles purchased to transport individuals who use wheelchairs.

FORD MOBILITY MOTORING PROGRAM
(800) 952-2248   (800) 833-0312 (TTY)
FAX (800) 292-7842
www.ford.com/en/ourServices/specialBuyingPrograms/-
mobilityMotoringProgram/default.htm

This program funds assistive equipment conversion up to $1000. Provides toll-free information line, FREE video that describes the program, list of assessment centers that determine equipment needs, and referrals to sources for additional assistance.

GENERAL MOTORS MOBILITY ASSISTANCE CENTER
100 Renaissance Center, PO Box 100
Detroit, MI 48265
(800) 323-9935   (800) 833-9935 (TTY)
www.gm.com/automotive/vehicle_shopping/gm_mobility

This program reimburses customers up to $1000 for vehicle modifications or adaptive driving devices for new or demo vehicles. Includes alerting devices for drivers who are deaf or hearing impaired, such as emergency vehicle siren detectors and enhanced turn signal reminders.

GREYHOUND LINES, INC.
PO Box 660362
Dallas, TX 75266-0362
(800) 231-2222 (General Information)
(800) 752-4841 (ADA Assist Line)
(800) 345-3109 (TTY)   www.Greyhound.com

Provides assistance to travelers with disabilities upon request. Call ADA Assist line at least 48 hours in advance of travel. Information also available on web site; click on "Travel Planning for Passengers with Disabilities."

INTERNAL REVENUE SERVICE (IRS)
(800) 829-1040   (800) 829-4059 (TTY)
www.irs.gov

The IRS provides technical assistance about tax credits and deductions related to accommodations for disabilities. To request Publication 502, "Medical and Dental Expenses," call (800) 829-3676; (800) 829-4059 (TTY). These publications are available on the web site.

MOSSREHAB RESOURCENET
www.mossresourcenet.org

This web site offers information on accessible travel for individuals with disabilities. Click on "Accessible Travel."

NATIONAL MOBILITY EQUIPMENT DEALERS ASSOCIATION
11211 North Nebraska Avenue, Suite A-5
Tampa, FL 33612
(800) 833-0427   (813) 977-6603
FAX (813) 977-6402   www.nmeda.org

The members of this organization are car dealers, manufacturers, driver evaluators, and insurance companies. Provides local referrals to members who are adaptive equipment dealers and rates members' competencies in equipment installation and conversion.

NATIONAL PARK SERVICE
U.S. Department of the Interior, Office of Public Affairs
1849 C Street, NW, Room 3045
Washington, DC 20240
(202) 208-6843   www.nps.gov

Operates the Golden Access Passport program for people who have disabilities. FREE brochure.

PROJECT ACTION ACCESSIBLE TRAVELER'S DATABASE
www.projectaction.org/paweb/index.htm

This database offers information on accessible transportation services, including accessible car and van rental companies, rural and urban transit operators, major hotel chains, and national toll-free numbers.

SOCIETY FOR ACCESSIBLE TRAVEL AND HOSPITALITY
347 Fifth Avenue, Suite 610
New York, NY 10016
(212) 447-7284   FAX (212) 725-8253
www.sath.org

Advocates for accessibility for individuals with disabilities and serves as a clearinghouse for information on barrier-free travel. Membership, individuals, $45.00; seniors and students, $30.00; includes quarterly newsletter, "Open World for Accessible Travel." FREE sample of newsletter is available on request.

TRANSPORTATION SECURITY ADMINISTRATION (TSA)
U.S. Department of Transportation
400 Seventh Street, SW
Washington, DC 20590
www.tsa.gov

Created by Congress under the Transportation Security Act, passed after the attack on the World Trade Center on September 11, 2001, this agency is responsible for establishing regulations to enhance passenger security related to all types of transportation. The web site has information specific to travelers who have disabilities.

UNITED STATES GOLF ASSOCIATION (USGA)
PO Box 708
Far Hills, NJ 07931-0708
(908) 234-2300   www.usga.org

The association's web site lists golf programs for individuals with disabilities. Also provides "A Modification of The Rules of Golf for Golfers with Disabilities," including those who are blind or visually impaired or have mobility impairments.

VSA ARTS
1300 Connecticut Avenue, NW, Suite 700
Washington, DC 20036
(800) 933-8721   (202) 737-0645 (TTY)
FAX (202) 737-0725   www.vsarts.org

Provides opportunities for individuals with disabilities to participate in fine and performing arts.

WHEELERS ACCESSIBLE VAN RENTAL
(800) 456-1371   www.wheelerz.com

Rents mini-vans accessible to wheelchair users throughout the country.

PUBLICATIONS

ACCESSIBLE GARDENING FOR PEOPLE WITH PHYSICAL DISABILITIES
by Janeen R. Adil
Woodbine House
6510 Bells Mill Road
Bethesda, MD 20817
(800) 843-7323   FAX (301) 897-5838
www.woodbinehouse.com

Written for people with a variety of mobility impairments, this book provides information on making existing gardens more accessible and creating new gardens. Sources for obtaining supplies are included. $16.95

ACCESS TO RECREATION
8 Sandra Court
Newbury Park, CA 91320
(800) 634-4351   (805) 498-7535
FAX (805) 498-8186   www.accesstr.com

Sells assistive devices that help people with disabilities enjoy sports and recreational activities, such as swimming aids, fishing equipment, fitness equipment and home gyms, golf clubs, wheelchair ramps, bowling aids, and adapted games.

ACCESS TRAVEL: AIRPORTS
Federal Consumer Information Center
PO Box 100
Pueblo, CO 81002
(888) 878-3256   www.pueblo.gsa.gov

This brochure lists facilities and services for people with disabilities in airport terminals worldwide. FREE. Also available on the web site.

THE DISABLED DRIVER'S MOBILITY GUIDE
c/o Kay Hamada, Traffic Safety and Engineering
American Automobile Association (AAA)
1000 AAA Drive
Heathrow, FL 32746
(407) 444-7961   FAX (407) 444-7956

This book provides information about adaptive equipment, driver training, and travel information services. $8.95

LARGE PRINT PUBLISHING COMPANY
103 Forest Glen
West Springfield, MA 01089
(800) 810-2777   FAX (413) 731-9156

Publishes LARGE PRINT puzzles, including crosswords, trivia, circle word puzzles, and adult coloring designs. Sample pack, $5.50.

NEW HORIZONS FOR THE AIR TRAVELER WITH A DISABILITY
Federal Consumer Information Center
PO Box 100
Pueblo, CO 81002
(888) 878-3256   www.pueblo.gsa.gov

This booklet provides information about the Air Carrier Access rules and other regulations that affect air travelers. FREE. Also available on the web site.

SOURCES OF INGENIOUS AIDS AND DEVICES

Suppliers of personal and home health care aids, recreational products, and mobility aids for more than one type of condition or disability are listed. For suppliers of aids and devices for a specific disability or condition, refer to the chapter that deals with that disability or condition (e.g., vision loss, hearing loss, etc.). Many hospital pharmacies as well as large department and discount stores now sell home health products such as wheelchairs, bathroom safety devices, canes, and walkers.

The following vendors sell assistive devices that help elders remain independent. Those that specialize in a specific type of product have a notation under the listing. Otherwise, their product line is broad, usually including personal, health care, and recreation aids and devices for the home. Unless otherwise noted, the catalogues are FREE.

Several guidebooks that provide tips and techniques for everyday living with a disability are also listed, as well as a quarterly magazine.

DYNAMIC LIVING, INC.
1265 John Fitch Boulevard, #9
South Windsor, CT 06074
(888) 940-0605   FAX (860) 291-8884
www.dynamic-living.com

ENRICHMENTS
Sammons Preston
PO Box 5071
Bolllingbrook, IL 60440
(800) 323-5547   FAX (800) 547-4333
www.sammonspreston.com

INDEPENDENT LIVING AIDS, INC.
200 Robbins Lane
Jericho, NY 11753
(800) 537-2118   FAX (516) 752-3135
www.independentliving.com

LS & S GROUP
PO Box 673
Northbrook, IL 60065
(800) 468-4789   (847) 498-1482
www.lssgroup.com

**MEALTIME MANUAL FOR PEOPLE WITH DISABILITIES AND
AGING**
by Judith L. Klinger
Slack Incorporated
6900 Grove Road
Thorofare, NJ 08086
(856) 848-1000   FAX (856) 853-5991
www.slackinc.com

This book provides information on meal planning and preparation
for individuals with mobility and visual impairments. Includes
hands-on skills and suggests many assistive devices. $25.95

MEDIC ALERT
PO Box 1009
Turlock, CA 95381
(800) 432-5378   In CA, (209) 668-3333
FAX (209) 669-2495   www.medicalert.org

Medical identification bracelet for people with serious medical
conditions.

RADIO SHACK/TANDY CORPORATION
500 One Tandy Center, 100 Throckmorton Street
Fort Worth, TX 76102
(817) 390-3700   www.radioshack.com

Radio Shack products for individuals with disabilities, such as talking watches and clocks and assistive listening aids, are included in the company's regular catalogues.

SEARS HEALTHCARE
7700 Brush Hill Road
Hinsdale, IL 60521
(800) 326-1750   (800) 733-7249 (TTY)

Sells health care and rehabilitation products.

SPECIALIVING MAGAZINE
PO Box 1000
Bloomington, IL 61072-1000
(888) 372-3737   (309) 825-8842
www.SpeciaLiving.com

This quarterly magazine features information on accessible housing, recreation, and aids for everyday living. $12.00

Chapter 4

ARTHRITIS

Arthritis is the term used to describe more than one hundred different conditions which cause aching and pain in joints and connective tissue. It is the most common cause of pain, disability, and disfigurement in the United States and affects people of all ages. Its prevalence among elders, however, is especially high. In 1996, 49% of elders reported that they had arthritis (Administration on Aging: 2001). The cause of arthritis is unknown, but scientists suspect that a virus may trigger the inflammatory process that affects joints and that some individuals may have an inherited susceptibility to the virus.

OSTEOARTHRITIS is the most common type of arthritis in elders. It is a chronic, nonsystemic, noninflammatory form of arthritis which results in the breakdown of the cartilage that covers the ends of the bones and other joint tissue. Age is a major risk factor in the development of osteoarthritis, and it is more common in women over the age of 54 than in men in the same age group (Arthritis Foundation: 1994). Genetic factors are thought responsible for about 50% of osteoarthritis of the hips and hands. Arthritis is diagnosed through physical examination, blood tests, urinalysis, x-rays, tests of joint fluids, or biopsy of muscle or joint tissue. Osteoarthritis does not affect the entire body but most commonly occurs in the joints of the fingers, hips, and knees, and the discs of the spine. Osteoarthritis may develop gradually, resulting in mild to severe disability.

The most common signs of osteoarthritis are painful bony growths in the joints of the fingers. It is a degenerative disease, formerly thought to be related to the overuse and abuse of joints through the "wear and tear" of aging. Actually, activity seems to protect joints. Lorig and Fries (1990) report that studies of individuals engaged in activities that put stress on joints, such as long distance running and the operation of pneumatic drills, are at no greater risk for osteoarthritis than those who do not engage in these activities. Obesity is a far greater risk factor for osteoarthritis of the knee. The Arthritis Foundation (1994) reports that controlling or losing weight may reduce this risk, citing a study in which women who lost as little as 11 pounds over a ten year span halved their risk for osteoarthritis of the knee. Osteoarthritis is a major indication for hip replacement surgery, which may result in functional improvement and relief of pain.

Osteoarthritis may exist simultaneously with other forms of the disease. It may also cause complications in the management of other chronic impairments and diseases. For example, when people with insulin-dependent diabetes also have arthritis, it may be difficult to grasp a syringe. Osteoarthritis may also affect rehabilitation for other health conditions, such as a stroke, when pain interferes with adaptive mobility techniques. Other conditions related to arthritis, such as bursitis, tendonitis, and fibrositis, involve inflammation or irritation of the muscles, tendons, and ligaments.

The Osteoarthritis Initiative (OAI), established in 2001, is a collaborative partnership between federal agencies, such as the National Institute on Aging and the National Institute of Arthritis and Musculoskeletal and Skin Diseases, and the pharmaceutical industry. A network of clinical centers will recruit individuals who are over age 50 and at high risk of having osteoarthritis to collect data on disease progression. It is hoped that the data, biological specimens, and imaging studies will lead to the discovery of biochemical markers and the development of promising treatments.

TREATMENT OF OSTEOARTHRITIS

Osteoarthritis treatment usually includes medication; rest; application of heat and/or cold; protection of joints with splints; weight-reduction to reduce joint strain; surgery to repair or replace damaged joints; and special exercises.

most common medications used to treat osteoarthritis by pain are analgesics and nonsteroidal anti-inflammatory (NSAIDs). Researchers who have compared these two _tions found that there was no difference in the relief of symptoms, although NSAIDS are more expensive and have greater risk of side effects (Brandt: 1993). Side effects of treatment with NSAIDs include stomach irritation, constipation, nausea, fluid retention, dizziness, and blood clotting problems. According to the Arthritis Foundation (1996), being female confers a greater risk of developing an ulcer while taking NSAIDs. Additional ulcer risk factors are age (over 60), a history of ulcers, use of corticosteroids, the presence of another chronic disease, drinking alcohol, and smoking. NSAIDs such as ibuprofen and naproxen are similar to aspirin but may have fewer side effects, although they have been implicated in gastrointestinal bleeding and renal problems (Fenner: 1992). It is recommended that these drugs be taken with meals in order to reduce stomach irritation.

Aspirin is a salicylate, a subcategory of NSAIDS, that may also cause gastrointestinal problems and bleeding tendencies and affect kidney function.

Cox-2 inhibitors are a new subcategory of NSAIDS claimed to reduce arthritis pain and inflammation without the gastrointestinal (GI) side effects of traditional NSAIDS. Celecoxib (Celebrex) was approved by the Food and Drug Administration (FDA) in 1998 for use by individuals with osteoarthritis and rheumatoid arthritis. After reports of bleeding complications in patients who also take warfarin, an anticoagulant used in the treatment of heart disease and stroke, it was recommended that these individuals be monitored to determine whether adjustment in the warfarin dose is needed. In 2002, after a long-term safety study, the FDA mandated that the geriatric section of celecoxib labeling warn of the risk of serious gastrointestinal and renal effects in elders (Food and Drug Administration: 2002). Rofecoxib (Vioxx) was approved in 1999 for use by individuals with osteoarthritis for the relief of pain.

Chemically modified salicylates, or nonacetylated salicylates, are usually safer and do not increase bleeding tendencies. Drugs in this category include choline salicylate (Arthropan), choline magnesium trisalicylate (Trilisate), and salsalate (Disalcid).

Analgesics may be prescribed to reduce pain when there is little inflammation. Acetaminophen is the most common analgesic. It is available in generic and brand-name (Anacin, Excedrin, Tylenol) forms. Narcotic analgesics (Darvon, Ultram) may be used for severe and chronic pain. Individuals who have swallowing problems should ask their physicians or pharmacists if liquid forms of these medications are available. A hollow handled medicine spoon is useful when taking these liquids.

Topical analgesics are creams or salves, such as BenGay, Zostrix, Capzasin-P, or Icy Hot, which are rubbed on to affected areas to stimulate or irritate nerve endings, distracting attention from musculoskeletal pain.

The Food and Drug Administration (FDA) has approved two drugs for treating osteoarthritis of the knee, hyaluronan (Hyalgan) and hylan G-F20 (Synvisc), which are injected into the knee joint to reduce the pain that occurs when joint fluid breaks down due to this disease. Relief lasts between six and 12 months.

Glucosamine sulfate and chondroitin sulfate, popular alternative therapies used by many individuals with arthritis, are approved as drugs in Europe and South America, but are available as dietary supplements only in the United States. Advocates claim that glucosamine stimulates growth and maintains the strength of cartilage. The National Institutes of Health is currently conducting clinical trials of both supplements.

The chronic, painful nature of osteoarthritis leads many people to fall prey to claims for quick cures or "miracle" drugs, which may not only harm the individual but also delay proper treatment.

More than 650,000 Americans undergo knee arthroscopy each year in the hope of alleviating the pain of osteoarthritis (Owings and Kozak: 1998). In this procedure, the orthopedic surgeon flushes the knee joint with fluid to remove loose debris, repairs tears, or smoothes rough cartilage. A recent randomized, placebo-controlled trial designed to measure the efficacy of this procedure reports that patients who underwent the procedure had no less pain or better function that those who had placebo surgery (Moseley et al.: 2002).

Knee replacement surgery has become more common and successful in recent years. Maintaining a healthy weight and exercising daily will contribute to post-surgical success. Elders contemplating surgery must also be evaluated for their ability and motivation to participate in a long postoperative rehabilitation program. Elders should investigate the benefits of joint replacement surgery very carefully, seeking more than one opinion, and taking their time in making a decision. The complication rate of knee replacement surgery is reduced when surgeons are experienced in the procedure and operate at facilities where at least 40 procedures are performed each year (Kass-Bartelmes: 2002).

Severe osteoarthritis in the hip may require total hip replacement surgery, to restore function and relieve pain. Since total hip replacements last an average of 15 years (Lorig and Fries: 1990), it is important to think about facing the pain, risk, and costs of repeating the procedure. It is wise to participate in a rehabilitation program following this surgery. Physical and occupational therapy services may be provided at a rehabilitation center, outpatient clinic, or in the home.

Because aspirin treatment may interfere with blood clotting factors, it should be discontinued at least a week before surgery to avoid bleeding during surgery and postoperatively. Individuals should consider giving their own blood prior to surgery so that it is available if needed during or after the operation. It may be wise to start performing exercises that will help with recovery. A physical therapist should be consulted before engaging in such an exercise program.

The role of exercise in increasing endurance for individuals with osteoarthritis is currently receiving increased attention.

Jurisson (1991) reports that a decrease in symptoms is an unexpected benefit of exercises such as walking, aquatics, and riding a stationary bicycle. Elders with arthritis benefit from a daily routine combining strengthening, range of motion, and endurance exercises followed by rest and relaxation. Range of motion exercises strengthen joints and reduce the loss of physical functioning. Walking and swimming help maintain flexible joints and also provide aerobic exercise that is good for the entire body and the sense of well-being. Swimming is particularly good for individuals whose knees and hips are affected. Exercise in the water reduces the stress on these major joints while increasing cardiovascular health and endurance.

A program of physical therapy may include heat and cold treatments, massage, and relaxation training to make the individual with osteoarthritis as comfortable as possible. Heat treatments may include hot baths or showers, hot packs, heat lamps, electric pads or mitts, paraffin wax applications, or blown hot air. Cold compresses or ice bags may also be effective. Transcutaneous electrical nerve stimulation (TENS) may be used to relieve pain. To protect joints, the physical therapist may recommend the use of canes, walkers, or crutches to reduce the body's weight on joints. Elders may also be taught to use their joints more safely; for example, pushing with the whole arm or side of the body rather than with the hand only. Splints or orthotics, which are devices used for support and to improve function in movable parts of the body, may be prescribed to stabilize weak joints and prevent them from becoming permanently stiff or bent. The physical therapist may also recommend rest to relieve inflammation and pain, although too much rest may lead to stiffness and poor joint movement. It is necessary to balance rest during flare-ups and activity during remissions.

PSYCHOLOGICAL ASPECTS OF OSTEOARTHRITIS

Pain is the major manifestation of osteoarthritis; therefore, pain management is a prime concern for elders and health care professionals. Progressive inactivity may result from pain coupled with diminishing vision, hearing loss, or other chronic conditions (Rudd and Katz: 1988). Elders who fear disability due to osteoarthritis may delay seeking treatment, placing themselves at greater risk for potential damage. Elders with osteoarthritis must learn how to cope with pain and to optimize their medical treatment program. It is important for the physician to explain these aspects of osteoarthritis to the individual.

When osteoarthritis makes work and activities of daily living difficult, it may affect interpersonal relationships both on the job and at home. If the individual is tired, in pain, or unable to move about easily, he or she may experience emotional problems such as depression, loss of self-esteem, and worry, which in turn make everyday life even more difficult. These problems combined with role reversal and mood changes due to medication may also lead to sexual dysfunction (Gerber: 1988); when osteoarthritis affects the hips, sexual activity may become painful. After hip replacement surgery, elders should ask their physicians when they may resume sexual activity. In addition to bedrest and joint rest, elders with osteoarthritis should make time for emotional rest. The Arthritis Foundation recommends learning stress reduction or relaxation techniques and participating in recreational activities and social groups.

The desire to remain independent provides strong motivation for rehabilitation. Patient education programs offered by hospitals, universities, Arthritis Foundation chapters, and senior centers teach self-management skills to elders in order to help them live as independently as possible. These courses often result in reduction in pain, dependency, and depression (National Resource Center on Health Promotion and Aging: 1989). Common topics in these courses are education about arthritis, exercise, emotional support, and discussions of how elders can advocate for themselves within the health care system and participate in choosing treatment options. The Arthritis Foundation offers a six week self-help course, which has been found to increase participants' perception of their own control over the disease, which in turn improves their health status (Haggerty: 1995). Online courses are also available on the Arthritis Foundation web site.

PROFESSIONAL SERVICE PROVIDERS

Services for elders with osteoarthritis are provided by a variety of health care professionals. In addition, voluntary organizations provide information, education, and support groups for elders.

RHEUMATOLOGISTS are physicians who specialize in the treatment of rheumatic diseases, which are inflammations and degenerations of joints and connective tissues.

ORTHOPEDIC SURGEONS or PLASTIC SURGEONS may perform surgery to repair or replace joints damaged by arthritis. Hip and knee replacement surgery may be recommended.

PHYSIATRISTS, physicians who specialize in rehabilitation medicine, often act as case managers or team leaders, coordinating medical and rehabilitation services, working with the elder with arthritis and the family, and arranging additional health care services if necessary.

PHYSICAL THERAPISTS develop an exercise program to control some arthritis symptoms; keep joints flexible; build up and preserve muscle strength; and help protect joints from further stress.

OCCUPATIONAL THERAPISTS teach the individual new techniques to perform everyday activities, such as washing and dressing, homemaking, and recreation. Many assistive devices, such as reaching tools, built-up kitchen utensils, and writing aids are suggested by the occupational therapist.

WHERE TO FIND SERVICES

The health care professionals who provide services to elders with osteoarthritis work in hospitals, rehabilitation centers, home health agencies, private and public agencies, independent living centers, and as private practitioners. Individual and group counseling may be available through a local hospital, community health center, senior center, or from mental health professionals in private practice. The Arthritis Foundation offers arthritis classes to help individuals understand and cope with their condition. Members of self-help groups share emotional support and practical advice. Some individuals attend pain clinics which teach behavior modification techniques to limit the effect of pain.

Elders who are severely disabled by osteoarthritis often require home health services such as home treatment and maintenance care. These services are provided by nurses or home health aides; special homemaker services; Meals on Wheels programs; chore services such as housecleaning; and adult day activity programs. The services are often FREE to low income elders, or the fees may be on a sliding scale.

When individuals with osteoarthritis require hospitalization for surgery, they may choose a rehabilitation unit within a community hospital or a rehabilitation hospital. Most rehabilitation centers also offer post-surgical outpatient services.

ASSISTIVE DEVICES AND
ENVIRONMENTAL ADAPTATIONS

Many elders with disabilities use assistive devices to make everyday living easier. These devices may be specially designed or they may be common items found in medical supply or hardware stores. They may be purchased in local stores or through mail-order catalogues. Schweidler (1984) identifies four basic functions of assistive devices for people with arthritis: to compensate for lost function; to alleviate joint stress; to decrease energy demands; and to increase safety.

The physical therapist or occupational therapist may recommend that the individual use an assistive device only at times when functioning is difficult. Individuals with arthritis must keep their joints flexible yet protect them from stress. It is also important to learn to use the assistive device correctly to avoid stress on other joints.

Many elders are familiar with devices such as can and jar openers; these simple tools compensate for a weak grasp. Long-handled tongs, utensils with built-up handles, and other adapted equipment will make it easier for the individual to continue home-making activities. Touch-sensitive lamps are controlled with a pat of the hand. A pen with a thick barrel is easier for individuals with arthritis to use than a slim-line design, because it reduces stress on finger joints. Dressing aids such as button hooks, elastic shoe laces, or zipper pulls, and clothing with velcro fasteners, elastic waistbands, or snaps enable the individual to conserve energy when dressing. It is easier to open and close doors when doorknobs are replaced with levers and push locks and push-pull latches are installed. Swing clear hinges on doors provide the clearance to accommodate wheelchairs and walkers. Adjustable height sinks and toilets are valuable additions in the bathroom as are grab bars for safety in the tub or shower. A cane may help the individual walk more safely by promoting balance. Battery-powered chairs or scooters help individuals who cannot walk long distances or stand for long periods of time continue activities, such as visiting museums and attending sports events. Elders with osteoarthritis also use assistive devices for recreational activities such as playing cards and gardening. Cardholders enable the individual to continue playing favorite card games and socializing with friends. Gardening tools are adapted with extension handles to reduce bending or built-up handles to make grasping easier. Individuals may ask their pharmacy to use non-childproof caps on medications for easier opening.

Special van services or special parking placards for people with disabilities may help solve some of the transportation problems of elders with arthritis. Architectural adaptations such as ramps, railings, chairlifts, and elevators may make independent mobility easier.

Although most assistive devices are nonprescription items, some may be covered by third-party payment with prior approval. (See Chapter 3, "MAKING EVERYDAY LIVING SAFER AND EASIER")

REFERENCES

Administration on Aging
2001 A PROFILE OF OLDER AMERICANS: 2001 Washington, DC: U.S. Department of Health and Human Services
Arthritis Foundation
1996 ASPIRIN AND OTHER NSAIDS Atlanta, GA: The Arthritis Foundation
1994 OSTEOARTHRITIS Atlanta, GA: The Arthritis Foundation
Brandt, Kenneth D.
1994 "Osteoarthritis" pp. 1692-1698 in Kurt J. Isselbacher et al. (eds.) HARRISON'S PRINCIPLES OF INTERNAL MEDICINE New York, NY: McGraw Hill
Fenner, Helmut
1992 "Nonsteroidal Anti-inflammatory Drugs: Benefit/Risk Evaluation in Rheumatic Diseases" JOURNAL OF RHEUMATOLOGY 19:(Supplement 32):98-99
Food and Drug Administration
2002 "Labeling Changes for Arthritis Drug Celebrex" FDA TALK PAPER June 7

Gerber, Lynn H.
1988 "Rehabilitative Therapies for Patients with Rheumatic Disease" pp. 301-307 in H. Ralph Schumacher, Jr. (ed.) PRIMER ON THE RHEUMATIC DISEASES Atlanta, GA: Arthritis Foundation

Haggerty, Maureen
1995 "Taking Control" ADVANCE/REHABILITATION 4(January)6:35-38

Jurisson, Mary L.
1991 "Rehabilitation in Rheumatic Diseases What's New" WESTERN JOURNAL OF MEDICINE 154:5:545-548

Kass-Bartelmes, Barbara L.
2002 "Managing Osteoarthritis: Helping the Elderly Maintain Function and Mobility" RESEARCH IN ACTION Rockville, MD: Agency for Healthcare Research and Quality

Lorig, Kate and James F. Fries
1990 THE ARTHRITIS HELPBOOK Reading, MA: Addison-Wesley Publishing Company

Moseley, J. Bruce et al.
2002 "A Controlled Trial of Arthroscopic Surgery for Osteoarthritis of the Knee" NEW ENGLAND JOURNAL OF MEDICINE 347:2(July 11):81-88

National Resource Center on Health Promotion and Aging
1989 "Arthritis: Positive Approaches Offer New Hope" PERSPECTIVES IN HEALTH PROMOTION AND AGING 4:(November-December)6

Owings, M.F. and L.J. Kozak
1998 "Ambulatory and Inpatient Procedures in the United States: 1996" NATIONAL CENTER FOR HEALTH STATISTICS Vital Health Statistics 13(139)

Rudd, Emmanuel and Warren Katz
1988 "Rehabilitation in Geriatric Rheumatology" pp. 184-199 in Jeanne F. Hicks et al. (eds.) HANDBOOK OF REHABILITATIVE RHEUMATOLOGY Atlanta, GA: American Rheumatism Association

Schweidler, Helen

1984   "Assistive Devices, Aids to Daily Living" pp. 263-276 in Gail Kershner Riggs and Eric P. Gall (eds.) RHEUMATIC DISEASES, REHABILITATION AND MANAGEMENT Boston, MA: Butterworth

ORGANIZATIONS

AMERICAN ACADEMY OF ORTHOPAEDIC SURGEONS
6300 North River Road
Rosemont, IL 60018
(800) 346-2267   (847) 823-7186
FAX (847) 823-8125   orthoinfo.aaos.org

A professional organization for orthopaedic surgeons and allied health professionals. Web site offers a "Find a Surgeon" link. The "Surgery Center" link provides information on types, benefits, and risks of surgery as well as preparing for surgery, hospitalization, and recovery. Surgery animations demonstrate procedures such as arthroscopy and hip, knee, and shoulder replacements. Fact sheets that relate to surgery and arthritis are available on the web site. A quarterly e-mail newsletter, "Your Orthopaedic Connection," is available upon request.

AMERICAN CHRONIC PAIN ASSOCIATION (ACPA)
PO Box 850
Rocklin, CA 95677
(916) 632-0922   FAX (916) 632-3208
www.theacpa.org

Organizes groups throughout the U.S. to provide support and activities for people who experience chronic pain. $30.00 first year, $15.00 thereafter; includes quarterly newsletter, "ACPA Chronicle."

AMERICAN COLLEGE OF RHEUMATOLOGY
1800 Century Place, Suite 250
Atlanta, GA 30345
(404) 633-3777   FAX (404) 633-1870
www.rheumatology.org

A professional membership organization for rheumatologists who treat or study all forms of arthritis. Will provide a list of rheumatologists in a single state. Offers fact sheets on rheumatic diseases such as osteoarthritis, rheumatoid arthritis, and gout. FREE. Also available on the web site.

AMERICAN PAIN FOUNDATION (APF)
201 North Charles Street, Suite 710
Baltimore, MD 2120
(888) 615-7246   FAX (410) 385-1832
www.painfoundation.org

This organization provides educational materials and advocates on behalf of people who are experiencing pain. Promotes research and advocates to remove barriers to treatment for pain. Distributes patient educational materials, FREE, and has information about the causes of pain and treatment as well as links to related sites on its web site.

ARTHRITIS CENTER
www.mayoclinic.com

This "Condition Center," found on the Mayo Clinic web site, provides information on many forms of arthritis as well as Healthy Lifestyle Planners for weight management, exercise, and stress management.

ARTHRITIS FOUNDATION
PO Box 7669
Atlanta, GA 30357-0669
(800) 283-7800   (404) 872-7100
FAX (404) 872-0457   www.arthritis.org

Supports research; offers referrals to physicians; provides public and professional education. Chapters throughout the U.S.; toll-free number connects to local chapter. Some chapters offer arthritis classes, clubs, and exercise programs. Membership, $20.00, includes chapter newsletter and magazine, "Arthritis Today." Also available by subscription, $12.95. Members receive discounts on purchases of publications. Many brochures are available on the web site. Several brochures are available in Spanish.

MEDLINEPLUS: OSTEOARTHRITIS
www.nlm.nih.gov/medlineplus/osteoarthritis.html

This web site provides links to sites for information about osteoarthritis, treatment, alternative therapy, clinical trials, disease management, specific conditions/aspects, everyday living, organizations, and research. Includes an interactive tutorial. Some information available in Spanish. Provides links to MEDLINE research articles and related MEDLINEplus pages.

NATIONAL CHRONIC PAIN OUTREACH ASSOCIATION (NCPOA)
PO Box 274
Millboro, VA 24460-9606
(540) 862-9437   FAX (540) 862-9485

A national clearinghouse for information about chronic pain. Refers individuals to support groups on chronic pain throughout the U.S. Produces publications and audiocassettes on a variety of topics related to chronic pain. Membership, individuals, $25.00; professionals, $50.00; includes quarterly newsletter, "Lifeline."

NATIONAL INSTITUTE OF ARTHRITIS AND MUSCULOSKELETAL AND SKIN DISEASES (NIAMS)
Building 31, Room 4C05
31 Center Drive, MSC 2350
Bethesda, MD 20892
(301) 496-8190   FAX (301) 480-2814
www.nih.gov/niams

Sponsors specialized research centers in osteoarthritis, rheumatoid arthritis, and osteoporosis. These centers conduct basic and clinical research; provide professional, public, and patient education; and are involved in community activities. Also supports individual clinical and basic research.

NATIONAL INSTITUTE OF ARTHRITIS AND MUSCULOSKELETAL AND SKIN DISEASES INFORMATION CLEARINGHOUSE (NAMSIC)
1 AMS Circle
Bethesda, MD 20892
(877) 226-4267   (301) 495-4484
(301) 565-2966 (TTY)   FAX (301) 718-6366
www.niams.nih.gov

Distributes bibliographies, fact sheets, catalogues, and directories to the public and professionals. FREE. Many of the fact sheets are available on the web site.

SPINE-HEALTH.COM
1840 Oak Avenue, Suite 112
Evanston, IL 60201
www.spine-health.com

This web site provides information on coping with chronic back pain, treatment, pain management, and rehabilitation. Also offers a physician directory on the web site.

PUBLICATIONS AND TAPES

THE ARTHRITIS ACTION PROGRAM
by Michael E. Weinblatt
Simon and Schuster
100 Front Street
Riverside, NJ 08075
(888) 866-6631   FAX (800) 943-9831
www.simonsays.com

This book describes common forms of arthritis, including osteoarthritis. Discusses treatment strategies, complementary therapies, exercises, pain management, and the role of physical and occupational therapists. $25.00

ARTHRITIS: A TAKE CARE OF YOURSELF HEALTH GUIDE
by James F. Fries
Perseus Books Group
Customer Service Department
5500 Central Avenue
Boulder, CO 80301
(800) 386-5656   www.perseuspublishing.com

This book describes major forms of arthritis and methods of managing the condition through exercise and new pain medications. Includes charts that help individuals make pain relief decisions. $16.00

THE ARTHRITIS HELPBOOK
by Kate Lorig and James J. Fries
Perseus Books Group
Customer Service Department
5500 Central Avenue
Boulder, CO 80301
(800) 386-5656   www.perseuspublishing.com

This book focuses on techniques that help reduce pain and increase dexterity. Includes information on prescription and over-the-counter medications, exercises, and nutrition. $19.00

ARTHRITIS OF THE HIP AND KNEE: THE ACTIVE PERSON'S GUIDE TO TAKING CHARGE
by Ronald J. Allen, Victoria Anne Brander, and S. David Stulberg
Peachtree Publishers
1700 Chattahoochee Avenue
Atlanta, GA 30324
(800) 241-0113   FAX (800) 875-8909
www.peachtree-online.com

This handbook, written by a patient who has had two hip replacements, an orthopedic surgeon, and a physiatrist, discusses the causes, treatment options, and progression of osteoarthritis. Includes information on hip replacement, post-operative physical therapy, the role of exercise, and advice on everyday activities. $14.95

CONNECT AND CONTROL
Arthritis Foundation
PO Box 7669
Atlanta, GA 30357-0669
(800) 283-7800   (404) 872-7100
FAX (404) 872-0457   www.arthritis.org

This online, interactive, self-management guide provides a personalized exercise program based on an individual's answers to a series of questionnaires. Weekly e-mails provide activities and information on additional topics such as nutrition, pain management, treatment options, emotional support, and managing stress and depression. FREE

COPING WITH OSTEOARTHRITIS
by Robert H. Phillips
Penguin Putnam, Inc.
(800) 788-6262   www.penguinputnam.com

Written by a psychologist, this book provides information for individuals and their families on coping with the condition and improving quality of life. $14.95

FEELING GOOD WITH ARTHRITIS
Info Vision
102 North Hazel Street
Glenwood, IA 51534
(800) 237-1808   FAX (888) 735-2622

This videotape discusses the importance of exercise, medical treatment, diet, and attitude. 60 minutes. $25.00

GUIDE TO GOOD LIVING WITH OSTEOARTHRITIS
Arthritis Foundation
PO Box 7669
Atlanta, GA 30357-0669
(800) 283-7800   (404) 872-7100
FAX (404) 872-0457   www.arthritis.org

This book provides information about the condition, its causes, and treatment. Includes practical tips for self-management. $16.95

LIVING AND LOVING: INFORMATION ABOUT SEX
Arthritis Foundation
PO Box 7669
Atlanta, GA 30357-0669
(800) 283-7800   (404) 872-7100
FAX (404) 872-0457   www.arthritis.org

This booklet discusses the effects that medication, physical problems, and emotional responses may have on sexuality in individuals with rheumatic diseases and their partners. Makes suggestions for improving sexual relations. $1.00

LIVING AT HOME WITH ARTHRITIS
A/V Health Services
PO Box 20271
Roanoke, VA 24018-0028
(540) 986-3275 (Voice and FAX)
www.avhealthservices.com

This videotape covers everyday activities, joint protection, and home modification and adaptive equipment. Includes stretching activities. 40 minutes. $70.00

MANAGING OSTEOARTHRITIS: HELPING THE ELDERLY MAINTAIN FUNCTION AND MOBILITY
Agency for Healthcare Research and Quality (AHRQ)
2101 East Jefferson Street, Suite 501
Rockville, MD 20852
(301) 594-1364   www.ahrq.gov

This report describes research that indicates that patient self-management, physical and occupational therapy, and surgery reduce the pain and functional disability of osteoarthritis. FREE. May be downloaded from the web site at no charge.

MANAGING YOUR ACTIVITIES
MANAGING YOUR FATIGUE
MANAGING YOUR HEALTH CARE
MANAGING YOUR PAIN
MANAGING YOUR STRESS
Arthritis Foundation
PO Box 7669
Atlanta, GA 30357-0669
(800) 283-7800   (404) 872-7100
FAX (404) 872-0457   www.arthritis.org

This series of brochures describes self-management techniques for coping with arthritis. "Managing Your Activities" suggests methods that will enable individuals to reduce stress on joints affected by arthritis and provides tips for self-help techniques and assistive devices. "Managing Your Fatigue" discusses fatigue, a common symptom in individuals with rheumatic disease. A "Fatigue Care Chart" enables individuals to identify causes of fatigue and suggests possible solutions. "Managing Your Health Care" describes the roles various health care professionals play in treating individuals with rheumatic diseases. Provides guidelines for making the most of office visits and a list of questions to ask physicians. "Managing Your Pain" discusses pain management strategies such as medication, exercise, assistive devices, heat and cold treatments, massage, and relaxation techniques. "Managing Your Stress" describes how stress can lead to physical and emotional reactions and discusses stress management techniques such as deep breathing, progressive relaxation, guided imagery, and visualization. Each brochure is $1.00.

OSTEOARTHRITIS
National Institute of Arthritis and Musculoskeletal and Skin Diseases Information Clearinghouse (NAMSIC)
1 AMS Circle
Bethesda, MD 20892
(877) 226-4267   (301) 495-4484
(301) 565-2966 (TTY)   FAX (301) 718-6366
www.niams.nih.gov

This booklet discusses the condition, diagnosis and treatment, pain relief, the role of exercise, and describes current research. FREE. Also available on the web site.

OSTEOARTHRITIS
Arthritis Foundation
PO Box 7669
Atlanta, GA 30357-0669
(800) 283-7800   (404) 872-7100
FAX (404) 872-0457   www.arthritis.org

This booklet describes the causes, diagnosis, and treatment of osteoarthritis. Includes "joint saver" tips to reduce pain. Available in English and Spanish. $1.00

OSTEOARTHRITIS AND RHEUMATOID ARTHRITIS
Films for the Humanities & Sciences
PO Box 2053
Princeton, NJ 08543-2053
(800) 257-5126   FAX (609) 275-3767
www.films.com

This videotape describes the differences between these two conditions as well as medical and surgical treatments. 19 minutes. Purchase, $99.95; one-day rental, $75.00.

OSTEOPOROSIS AND ARTHRITIS: TWO COMMON BUT DIFFERENT CONDITIONS
NIH Osteoporosis and Related Bone Diseases National Resource Center (ORBD)
1232 22nd Street, NW
Washington, DC 20037
(800) 624-2663   (202) 223-0344
(202) 466-4315 (TTY)   FAX (202) 223-2237
www.osteo.org

This brochure provides an overview of the risk factors, physical effects, treatment options, and pain management strategies associated with osteoporosis, osteoarthritis, and rheumatoid arthritis. FREE. Also available on the web site.

PATHWAYS TO BETTER LIVING WITH ARTHRITIS
PEOPLE WITH ARTHRITIS CAN EXERCISE (PACE)
POOL EXERCISE PROGRAM (PEP)
Arthritis Foundation
PO Box 7669
Atlanta, GA 30357-0669
(800) 283-7800   (404) 872-7100
FAX (404) 872-0457   www.arthritis.org

Videotape exercise programs developed by the Arthritis Foundation. "Pathways" demonstrates a wide variety of exercises for people of all ages and fitness levels; 55 minutes. "PACE Level 1" is a gentle exercise program for individuals with significant joint disease; 30 minutes. "PACE Level 2" is a moderate exercise program designed to increase endurance for individuals with mild arthritis; 40 minutes. "PEP" presents exercises to perform in chest level water. $19.50 each

QUESTIONS AND ANSWERS ABOUT ARTHRITIS PAIN

National Institute of Arthritis and Musculoskeletal and Skin Diseases Information Clearinghouse
1 AMS Circle
Bethesda, MD 20892
(877) 226-4267   (301) 495-4484
(301) 565-2966 (TTY)   FAX (301) 718-6366
www.niams.nih.gov

This booklet discusses short-term and long-term management of chronic arthritis pain, alternative therapies, and coping strategies. FREE. Also available on the web site.

QUESTIONS AND ANSWERS ABOUT HIP REPLACEMENT

National Institute of Arthritis and Musculoskeletal and Skin Diseases Information Clearinghouse
1 AMS Circle
Bethesda, MD 20892
(877) 226-4267   (301) 495-4484
(301) 565-2966 (TTY)   FAX (301) 718-6366
www.niams.nih.gov

This booklet discusses the surgical procedure, possible complications, recovery, and rehabilitation. FREE. Also available on the web site.

RECOVERING FROM HIP REPLACEMENT SURGERY

A/V Health Services
PO Box 20271
Roanoke, VA 24018-0028
(540) 986-3275 (Voice and FAX)
www.avhealthservices.com

This videotape follows an individual through a typical day following hip replacement surgery. Includes getting in and out of bed and car, using a walker and other adaptive equipment, and safety issues. 22 minutes. $70.00

TIPS FOR GOOD LIVING WITH ARTHRITIS
Arthritis Foundation
PO Box 7669
Atlanta, GA 30357-0669
(800) 283-7800   (404) 872-7100
FAX (404) 872-0457   www.arthritis.org

This guide provides practical tips for everyday activities and suggests assistive devices. $9.95

2002 DRUG GUIDE
Arthritis Foundation
PO Box 7669
Atlanta, GA 30357-0669
(800) 283-7800   (404) 872-7100
FAX (404) 872-0457   www.arthritis.org

This guide, published annually, reviews the drugs used in treating arthritis and related conditions. Includes a "Drug and Dosage Diary." FREE

RESOURCES FOR ASSISTIVE DEVICES

Listed below are publications that provide information about assistive devices and catalogues that specialize in devices for people with arthritis. Generic catalogues that sell some aids for people with arthritis are listed in Chapter 3, "MAKING EVERYDAY LIVING SAFER AND EASIER."

LIVING BETTER WITH ARTHRITIS
Aids for Arthritis, Inc.
35 Wakefield Drive
Medford, NJ 08055
(800) 654-0707   FAX (609) 654-8631
www.aidsforarthritis.com

A mail order catalogue of products with dressing, bathing, and grooming aids and kitchen, housekeeping, and recreation equipment. FREE. Also available on the web site.

SEARS HOME HEALTHCARE CATALOG
7700 Brush Hill Road
Hinsdale, IL 60521
(800) 326-1750   (800) 733-7249 (TTY)

Sells health care and rehabilitation products.

Chapter 5

DIABETES

Diabetes mellitus is a term that applies to a variety of disorders where the body is unable to maintain normal glucose levels. Hyperglycemia is a condition where the level of glucose in the blood is too high. Symptoms include extreme thirst, a dry mouth, excessive urination, blurred vision, lethargy and, in extreme cases, diabetic coma. If untreated, hyperglycemia can result in infections and poor wound healing (Henry and Edelman: 1992). Hypoglycemia is a condition where the level of glucose is too low. Symptoms may include feeling shaky or sweaty, headache, hunger, and dizziness. If untreated, hypoglycemia may result in angina, seizures, stroke, or myocardial infarction. Although there is no cure for diabetes, there are means to control the disease and to decrease the risk of the numerous associated complications. Early diagnosis and an intervention plan designed to meet the individual's specific needs are crucial steps in maintaining proper control of diabetes.

As the prevalence of diabetes has increased, it has become a major health problem in the United States and an important contributor to the cost of health care. From 1990 to 2000, the number of individuals with diagnosed diabetes increased 49% (Centers for Disease Control and Prevention: 2002). Over 10 million Americans age 20 or older, or 5.1% of the population, have been diagnosed with diabetes; an additional 5.4 million have the disease but have not been diagnosed (Harris et al.: 1998).

Diabetes is an age-related disease, occurring in 18.4% of those age 65 or over (Centers for Disease Control and Prevention: 1997a). African-Americans and Hispanics have higher rates of diabetes than whites. Unfortunately, the data sources for determining rates of diabetes among other minority groups are inadequate and do not provide accurate estimates. It is known that among Native Americans rates vary by tribe and that the Pima Indians of Arizona have the highest recorded prevalence - more than 50% of adults age 35 or over have diabetes (Centers for Disease Control and Prevention: 1997a). Over half of the elders who have diabetes have experienced limitations in their activity (Centers for Disease Control and Prevention: 1997a).

Diabetes and its complications are responsible for many hospital stays and have a large economic impact on society. Ng et al. (2001) found that individuals with diabetes lost about one-third of their annual earnings, due in large part to the complications caused by the disease.

Some observers believe that health professionals neglect diabetes among elders, since the more severe type usually occurs in the younger population (Tattersall: 1984). However, all forms of diabetes are serious, and elders are likely to have additional chronic diseases or impairments that affect their ability to control their diabetes. In fact, complications may develop quickly in elders who have actually had diabetes for a long period before it was diagnosed (National Diabetes Information Clearinghouse: 2002). A study (Testa and Simonson: 1998) found that even moderate improvements in glycemic control contributed to improved quality of life by decreasing fatigue and weakness as well as memory loss.

TYPES OF DIABETES

The two major types of diabetes mellitus are referred to as type 1 and type 2. In type 1 diabetes, the pancreas does not produce insulin, a substance that is necessary to metabolize the glucose (sugar) that the body needs for energy. Individuals with type 1 diabetes must take regular insulin injections to compensate. For this reason, type 1 is also referred to as insulin-dependent diabetes mellitus (IDDM). This variant of the disease is sometimes called juvenile-onset diabetes, because it usually is diagnosed at a young age. Approximately five to ten percent of Americans who have diabetes have type 1 (Centers for Disease Control and Prevention: 1997b).

In type 2 diabetes, the body produces some insulin but does not produce enough or does not utilize it properly. Because type 2 diabetes does not require insulin injections, it is also referred to as noninsulin-dependent diabetes mellitus (NIDDM). This type of the disease is often called adult-onset or maturity-onset diabetes, because most frequently it is diagnosed after age forty. It is estimated that over 90% of the cases of diabetes in the United States are type 2 (National Center for Health Statistics: 1987).

Although the causes of type 2 diabetes are not known, obesity and a family history of diabetes are predisposing factors. Symptoms of noninsulin-dependent diabetes, the type most common in elders, include fatigue, frequent urination, and excessive thirst. Elders who have these symptoms should make an appointment for a physical examination. However, diabetes is sometimes present when no symptoms are evident (Williams: 1983). In many cases, noninsulin-dependent diabetes can be controlled through both diet and exercise, although in some cases oral hypoglycemic agents are prescribed.

A subtype of diabetes caused by a defect in the mitochondrial DNA has recently been discovered. Called maternally inherited diabetes and deafness (MIDD) because the mitochondrial DNA is inherited only from the mother, this type of diabetes is associated with deafness and may be either type 1 or type 2 diabetes (Kobayashi et al.: 1997). In most cases, individuals with this type of diabetes are not obese. If they have type 2 diabetes, they usually do not need insulin in the early stages of the disease, although they may need it as the disease progresses. Protein in the urine, a sign of kidney disease, is sometimes diagnosed in individuals with MIDD; this clinical symptom is caused by the mutation, not the diabetes (Jansen et al.: 1997). A study of individuals with MIDD found that subjects treated with a dietary supplement, coenzyme Q10, had better outcomes in terms of beta cell production (the cells produced by the pancreas that are responsible for insulin production) and hearing than members of a control group (Suzuki et al.: 1998).

Diet and exercise for people with diabetes should be planned with a physician's advice to ensure that all medical conditions are taken into account. The goals of dietary restrictions are to reduce total body weight and to minimize the intake of glucose. Policy recommendations from the American Diabetes Association (1994) indicate that the use of simple sugars such as sucrose (table sugar) is not off limits and that they do not cause greater or more rapid rises in blood glucose than other carbohydrates. Scientific evidence suggests that sucrose has a similar effect on blood glucose as bread, rice, and potatoes. It is important to keep in mind the total amount of carbohydrates consumed and that simple sugars must be used in place of other carbohydrates in the diet. With the food labeling laws mandated by the federal government, this calculation becomes much easier, as the amount of carbohydrates per serving must be indicated on the food label. In order to control the amount of carbohydrates, many foods, including desserts and candies, are sweetened with artificial sweeteners.

Public libraries are a good source for the myriad cookbooks that have been written especially for people with diabetes. Discovering the variety of interesting recipes, including those for dessert and candies, should prove to be a psychological boost for elders who fear being restricted to bland meals.

A number of food manufacturers cater to the dietary needs of individuals with diabetes, and their products are often available in the dietetic food section of large supermarkets. Health food or natural food stores also carry many products that are amenable to the diet of people with diabetes. Perseverance in tracking down the right foods will allow for an interesting and varied diet; however, the shock and depression that follow the diagnosis of diabetes may limit the individual's emotional endurance. Support from a family member or close friend can help elders with diabetes to carry out this endeavor.

Exercise helps the body to use glucose and thus is an important part of the plan to control diabetes. After consulting with a physician, even elders who have been sedentary can begin a gradual exercise program by starting to take brief daily walks. When diet and exercise are insufficient to control type 2 diabetes, oral medications are prescribed. Sulfonylureas are a type of medication that causes the pancreas to produce increased amounts of insulin. Side effects of this type of medication include hypoglycemia and hyperinsulinemia, a condition in which too much insulin is in the bloodstream. Hyperinsulinemia is a risk factor for vascular disease and heart attack. In addition, sulfonylureas often fail to work after a number of years, causing the pancreas to fail. When this occurs, individuals must begin injecting insulin.

Several drugs that use different mechanisms to control diabetes have recently been approved by the Food and Drug Administration (FDA). One drug that has been available throughout much of the world since the late 1950s, metformin (Glucophage), was approved for use in the United States in 1995. Although it is not clear exactly how metformin works, it is effective in lowering blood glucose levels and has no serious side effects, unless the individual has kidney disease at the outset. Another drug approved by the FDA is acarbose, a carbohydrase inhibitor. Carbohydrases are the enzymes that break down carbohydrates and turn them into glucose. The side effects of acarbose are bloating, gas, and diarrhea, which may subside after six months of taking the drug.

Although testing urine for sugar was previously used to monitor glucose levels, this method is not as accurate as testing the blood directly. People with diabetes use home blood glucose monitoring equipment to measure glucose levels; this involves putting a drop of blood from a fingertip on a specially treated strip designed to react to the glucose. A digital display or speech output indicates the blood glucose level, and some monitors record the date and time of the reading. Illness, even a simple cold, can affect how the body uses insulin; glucose monitoring is even more important at these times. Log booklets enable individuals to keep a record of their blood glucose levels and to analyze their diets and schedules to determine what causes them to have varying levels of blood glucose. Home blood glucose monitors are inexpensive and are quite compact, making them suitable for use at home and when traveling. Some insurance companies pay for the cost of the test strips, although in some cases, only individuals who have insulin dependent diabetes receive this coverage. As of July 1, 1998, Medicare began paying for the cost of supplies for all beneficiaries who have diabetes, whether or not they take insulin. Supplies include blood glucose monitors, lancets, test strips, insulin, etc.

All types of diabetes have the same potential long term health effects. It is essential that elders with diabetes be aware of the proper management of their disease and all of the potential complications. Complications of diabetes include greater risks of heart disease, stroke, infections, and kidney disease (nephropathy); circulatory problems that can be especially problematic for legs and feet (resulting in amputation in extreme cases); neuropathy or nerve disease which causes tingling, numbness, double vision, pain, or dizziness; and vision problems.

Among the leading vision problems caused by diabetes is diabetic retinopathy. Visual impairment occurs when the small blood vessels in the retina are damaged and bleed inside the eye. If detected early, diabetic retinopathy can sometimes be treated successfully by laser therapy. In other cases, surgical procedures are performed in an attempt to restore useful vision. Individuals with diabetes should have regular examinations performed by ophthalmologists to detect any pathological conditions and receive appropriate treatment.

To manage their diabetes, many people with visual impairments use a wide range of adapted equipment such as blood glucose meters, scales, and thermometers with speech output; syringe magnifiers; and special insulin gauges. Special syringes that automatically measure insulin doses are useful for individuals with visual impairments as well as for those with arthritis or tremors. Sources for these aids are listed in the section titled "SPECIAL EQUIPMENT FOR PEOPLE WITH VISUAL IMPAIRMENTS" below.

The Diabetes Control and Complications Trial (1993) reported the results of a study which monitored 1,441 individuals with type 1 diabetes who were assigned to receive either conventional therapy (one or two injections of insulin daily) or intensive therapy (three or more injections of insulin daily). Results indicate that the intensive therapy group had significantly lower incidence of retinopathy, nephropathy, and neuropathy. The chief adverse effect of intensive therapy was increased episodes of severe hypoglycemia.

A British study carried out over a period of 20 years (UK Prospective Diabetes Study Group: 1998a) found that intensive control had similar benefits for individuals with type 2 diabetes. Individuals whose diabetes was controlled by sulfonylureas or insulin also had increased episodes of hypoglycemia. Obese individuals treated with metformin had even lower risks for diabetes complications and fewer episodes of hypoglycemia than individuals treated with sulfonylureas or insulin (UK Prospective Diabetes Study Group: 1998b).

A study by the Diabetes Prevention Program Research Group (2002) found that lifestyle changes that included exercise of at least 150 minutes per week and weight loss of seven percent reduced the incidence of type 2 diabetes among subjects whose blood glucose levels placed them at high risk for type 2 diabetes. Compared to a group that received a placebo, the group with lifestyle changes had a 58% lower incidence of type 2 diabetes. A third group that was treated with metformin had a 31% lower incidence of type 2 diabetes than the placebo group.

PSYCHOLOGICAL ASPECTS OF DIABETES

Although shock, fear, and depression are normal first reactions to the diagnosis of diabetes, a professional's careful explanation of the ability to control the disease can do much to alleviate these emotions. A common response to diabetes is a sense of loss of control over one's body. Because diabetes affects so many parts of the body, it also affects many aspects of daily life. In addition to prescribed changes in diet and exercise, elders with diabetes must always be aware of the symptoms that indicate hyperglycemia or hypoglycemia.

Changes in daily routines are never accepted readily. For elders, especially those who have other chronic impairments or diseases, changes in lifestyle and the need to monitor glucose may cause great stress. Social events and travel must be carefully planned to ensure that meals will comply with special diets. Glucose monitoring equipment must be packed for travel and regular monitoring activities carried out.

Another common response to type 2 diabetes is that "It's just a touch of diabetes." This response can be extremely dangerous when the individual fails to properly monitor and control the disease, because he or she does not understand its potential impact. Professionals should provide patients and family members with a frank explanation of the disease and its potential effects so that they understand the importance of the prescribed dietary regimen, exercise, and blood glucose monitoring. Professionals should not assume that elders are not capable of caring for themselves properly solely because of their age. Family members should also be instructed to allow elders to have the maximum possible responsibility for caring for themselves.

Although the effects of diabetes in elders vary greatly, service providers can help elders cope with their disease by providing educational information; inviting guest speakers on various aspects of diabetes; and sponsoring support groups for elders with diabetes and for family members. Those agencies that serve meals to elders should be certain that the food is healthy for individuals with diabetes.

Patients should understand their own responsibility for following the prescribed regimen to control diabetes, but they should not be made to feel guilty when their glucose is out of control. Diligent efforts to control glucose by following the recommended dosages of insulin or diets do not always result in the desired response. Individuals whose glucose is out of control should learn not to feel guilty; they may need to have their insulin or medication dosage and diet modified by a health care professional.

PROFESSIONAL SERVICE PROVIDERS

Because diabetes is a systemic disease, it has a wide range of effects. As a result, many types of health care professionals are involved in caring for people with diabetes. It is essential that these health care professionals provide coordinated care for patients, taking into account all of the patient's physical characteristics and conditions.

FAMILY PHYSICIANS and INTERNISTS are the physicians in charge of coordinating the various aspects of care for patients with diabetes. DIABETOLOGISTS are physicians who specialize in the treatment of individuals with diabetes.

NEPHROLOGISTS are physicians who treat people with kidney disease, which is a common complication of diabetes.

CERTIFIED DIABETES EDUCATORS (CDE) are health care professionals certified by the American Association of Diabetes Educators to teach individuals with diabetes how to effectively manage their disease. Although most CDEs are nurses or dietitians, they may be physicians, social workers, or other health care providers. They teach people with diabetes how to monitor their glucose levels, to modify their diets, care for their feet, and perform other activities essential to good management of diabetes.

OPHTHALMOLOGISTS are physicians who specialize in diseases of the eye. When diabetic retinopathy is present, patients are often referred to subspecialists called retina and vitreous specialists.

DIETITIANS or **NUTRITIONISTS** help people with diabetes plan a diet to control their blood glucose levels.

PHYSICAL THERAPISTS may help people with diabetes with their exercise regimen.

PSYCHOLOGISTS, SOCIAL WORKERS, and other counselors help people with diabetes and their family members adjust to the regimen prescribed to control the diabetes.

WHERE TO FIND SERVICES

In some areas, special treatment centers for diabetes and dialysis centers for people with kidney disease are available. The special physicians listed above practice in hospitals and also have private practices. Affiliates of the American Diabetes Association (ADA) exist in every state. These affiliates may provide publications, educational programs, and referrals to local resources. The national office (listed below under "ORGANIZATIONS") can provide the address and phone number of local affiliates. The ADA also has information about support groups that may be useful to elders. Understanding that other elders with diabetes continue to live fulfilling lives can be an extremely important benefit of attending support groups. Elders with diabetes who have vision problems may obtain services from public or private rehabilitation agencies serving individuals who are visually impaired or blind (see Chapter 10, "VISION LOSS").

ASSISTIVE DEVICES

Special equipment for elders with diabetes include prefilled syringes for injecting insulin, needle-free injectors, and devices for measuring insulin. Blood glucose monitors are necessary for both type 1 and type 2 forms of diabetes. These are usually prescribed by medical professionals, so this chapter will not go into detail about these devices. Since many people with diabetes have experienced visual impairments as a complication of their disease, they are often unable to use the standard versions of the necessary equipment. A section at the end of this chapter lists vendors of special equipment that enables elders with visual impairments to continue monitoring their disease.

REFERENCES

American Diabetes Association
1994 "Nutrition Recommendations and Principles for People with Diabetes Mellitus" DIABETES CARE 17(May)5:519-522
Centers for Disease Control
2002 DIABETES: DISABLING, DEADLY, ON THE RISE Atlanta, GA: Centers for Disease Control and Prevention
1997a DIABETES SURVEILLANCE 1997 Atlanta, GA: Public Health Service
1997b NATIONAL DIABETES FACT SHEET: NATIONAL ESTIMATES AND GENERAL INFORMATION ON DIABETES IN THE UNITED STATES Atlanta, GA: Centers for Disease Control and Prevention
Diabetes Control and Complications Trial Research Group
1993 "The Effect of Intensive Treatment of Diabetes on the Development and Progression of Long-Term Complications in Insulin-Dependent Diabetes Mellitus" NEW ENGLAND JOURNAL OF MEDICINE 329(September 30):14:977-986
Diabetes Prevention Program Research Group
2002 "Reduction in the Incidence of Type 2 Diabetes with Lifestyle Intervention or Metformin" NEW ENGLAND JOURNAL OF MEDICINE 346(February 7):393-403
Harris, Maureen I. et al.
1998 "Prevalence of Diabetes, Impaired Fasting Glucose, and Impaired Glucose Tolerance in U.S. Adults" DIABETES CARE 21:4(April):518-524
Henry, Robert R. and Steven V. Edelman
1992 "Advances in Treatment of Type II Diabetes Mellitus in the Elderly" GERIATRICS 47:4(April)24-30

Jansen, J.J. et al.

1997 "Mutation in Mitochondrial tRNA (Leu(UUR)) Gene Associated with Progressive Kidney Disease" JOURNAL OF THE AMERICAN SOCIETY OF NEPHROLOGY 8:7(July):1118-1124

Kobayashi, Tetsuro et al.

1997 "In Situ Characterization of Islets in Diabetes with a Mitochondrial DNA Mutation at Nucleotide Position 3243" DIABETES 46:1(October):1567-15710

National Center for Health Statistics

1987 "Health Practices and Perceptions of U.S. Adults with Noninsulin-dependent Diabetes. Data from the 1985 National Health Interview Survey of Health Promotion and Disease Prevention" ADVANCE DATA FROM VITAL AND HEALTH STATISTICS, No. 141, DHHS Pub. No. (PHS) 87-1250. Hyattsville, MD: Public Health Service, September 23, 1987

National Diabetes Information Clearinghouse

2002 "Diabetes and Aging" DIABETES DATELINE

Ng, Ying Chu, Philip Jacobs, and J.A. Johnson

2001 "Productivity Losses Associated with Diabetes in the U.S." DIABETES CARE 24:2(February):257-261

Suzuki, S. et al.

1998 "The Effects of Coenzyme Q10 Treatment on Maternally Inherited Diabetes and Deafness and Mitochondrial DNA 3243 (A to G) Mutation" DIABETOLOGIA 41:5(May):584-588

Tattersall, R.B.

1984 "Diabetes in the Elderly - A Neglected Area?" DIABETOLOGIA 27:167-173

Testa, Marcia and Donald Simonson

1998 "Health Economic Benefits and Quality of Life during Improved Glycemic Control in Patients with Type 2 Diabetes Mellitus" JAMA 280:17(November 4):1490-1496

UK Prospective Diabetes Study Group
1998a "Intensive Blood-Glucose Control with Sulphonylureas or Insulin Compared with Conventional Treatment and Risk of Complications in Patients with Type 2 Diabetes" THE LANCET 352(September 12):837-853
1998b "Effect of Intensive Blood-Glucose Control with Metformin on Complications in Overweight Patients with Type 2 Diabetes" THE LANCET 352(September 12):854-865
Williams, T. Franklin
1983 "Diabetes Mellitus in Older People" pp. 411-415 in William Reichel (ed.) CLINICAL ASPECTS OF AGING Baltimore, MD: Williams and Wilkins

ORGANIZATIONS

AMERICAN ASSOCIATION OF KIDNEY PATIENTS (AAKP)
3505 East Frontage Road, Suite 315
Tampa, FL 33607
(800) 749-2257   (813) 636-8100
FAX (813) 636-8122   www.aakp.org

Advocates on behalf of patients with kidney disease; sponsors local patient and family support groups; holds conferences and seminars. Membership, patients/families, $25.00; professionals, $35.00; includes quarterly newsletter, "aakpRENALIFE." Also available on the web site.

AMERICAN DIABETES ASSOCIATION (ADA)
1701 North Beauregard Street
Alexandria, VA 22311
(800) 342-2383
In the Washington, DC, (703) 549-1500
FAX (703) 836-7439   www.diabetes.org

National membership organization with local affiliates. Publications for both professionals and consumers, including cookbooks and guides for the management of diabetes (see "PUBLICATIONS AND TAPES" section below). Membership, $28.00, which includes membership in a local affiliate, discounts on publications, a subscription to "Diabetes Forecast" (Also available on cassette from the National Library Service. See Chapter 10, "VISION LOSS"). The January issue includes a resource guide to diabetes products. Many local affiliates offer their own publications, sponsor support groups, and conduct professional training programs. The web site includes featured articles from "Diabetes Forecast" and the medical journal "Diabetes Care" as well as basic information on diabetes. Publications ordered through the web site receive a discount. A toll-free hotline [(800)

342-2383)] offers information on diabetes and a packet of information.

AMERICAN DIETETIC ASSOCIATION (ADA)
216 West Jackson Boulevard
Chicago, IL 60606
(800) 877-1600   (312) 899-0040
FAX (312) 899-1758   www.eatright.org

Consumers may receive a referral to a registered dietitian or receive information about nutrition on the telephone or on the web site. Available in English and Spanish.

AMERICAN KIDNEY FUND
6110 Executive Boulevard, Suite 1010
Rockville, MD 20852
(800) 638-8299   (301) 881-3052
FAX (301) 881-0898   www.kidneyfund.org

Provides public and professional education and financial aid to individuals who have chronic kidney problems.

AMPUTEE COALITION OF AMERICA (ACA)
National Limb Loss Information Center
900 East Hill Avenue, Suite 285
Knoxville, TN 37915
(888) 267-5669   (865) 524-8772
FAX (865) 525-7917   www.amputee-coalition.org

Provides education and support services to individuals with amputations through a network of peer support groups, educational programs for health professionals, and a database of resources.   Membership, individuals, $25.00; professionals, $50.00; includes bimonthly magazine, "In-Motion."   Guides for organizing peer support groups and peer visitation programs also available.

CDC DIVISION OF DIABETES TRANSLATION
PO Box 8728
Silver Spring, MD 20910
(877) 232-3422   FAX (301) 562-1050
www.cdc.gov/diabetes

The Centers for Disease Control Division of Diabetes Translation conducts research related to the prevalence of diabetes; assesses clinical practices in order to develop optimal treatment; and works with state health departments to develop diabetes control programs.

DIABETES ACTION NETWORK
National Federation of the Blind
1412 I-70 Drive SW, Suite C
Columbia, MO 65203
(573) 875-8911   FAX (573) 875-8902
www.nfb.org/diabetes.htm

A national support and information network. Publishes a quarterly magazine, "Voice of the Diabetic," which includes personal experiences, medical information, recipes, and resources. Available in standard print, four-track audiocassette, and on the web site. Nonmembers may also obtain free subscriptions but are encouraged to pay $20.00. Also available, "Diabetes Resources: Equipment, Services and Information," a list of adaptive equipment; available in standard print and alternate formats, $5.00. Order from: National Federation of the Blind, 1800 Johnson Street, Baltimore, MD 21230. Also available on the web site.

DIABETES EXERCISE AND SPORTS ASSOCIATION (DESA)
formerly International Diabetic Athletes Association
PO Box 1935
Litchfield Park, AZ 85340
(800) 898-4322   (623) 535-4593
FAX (623) 535-4741   www.diabetes-exercise.org

An organization that provides education for individuals with diabetes who participate in sports and fitness activities, family members, and service providers through conferences, workshops, and publications. Membership, individuals, $30.00; corporate, $150.00; includes quarterly newsletter, "The Challenge."

DIABETES-SIGHT.ORG
www.diabetes-sight.org

Sponsored by Prevent Blindness America, this web site provides information for individuals and professionals about prevention of vision loss due to diabetes. Includes interactive tools such as a quiz, vision loss simulation, and tour of the eye's anatomy as well as research summaries and preferred practice guidelines for clinicians.

DIABETIC RETINOPATHY FOUNDATION
350 North LaSalle, Suite 800
Chicago, IL 60610
www.retinopathy.org

Supports research and public awareness in an effort to prevent diabetic retinopathy. Web site offers information about diabetic retinopathy and links to other web sites.

MEDLINEPLUS: DIABETES
www.nlm.nih.gov/medlineplus/diabetes.html

This web site provides links to sites for general information about diabetes, symptoms and diagnosis, treatment, alternative therapy, clinical trials, disease management, organizations, and research. Includes an interactive tutorial. Some information available in Spanish. Provides links to MEDLINE research articles and related MEDLINEplus pages.

NATIONAL DIABETES EDUCATION PROGRAM (NDEP)
National Institute of Diabetes and Digestive and Kidney Diseases (NIDDKD)
31 Center Drive, MSC 2560
Washington, DC 20892
(800) 438-5383   (301) 496-3583
www.ndep.nih.gov

A joint project of the National Institutes of Health and the Centers for Disease Control and Prevention, this program aims to prevent the increase in diabetes in this country through partnerships with other organizations that will provide public information about the disease. The web site has information about diabetes, and the program has produced public information materials, including cookbooks. FREE

NATIONAL DIABETES INFORMATION CLEARINGHOUSE (NDIC)
1 Information Way
Bethesda, MD 20892
(800) 860-8747   (301) 654-3327
FAX (301) 907-8906
www.niddk.nih.gov/health/diabetes/ndic.htm

Sponsored by the federal government, this clearinghouse publishes a variety of booklets related to diabetes. Titles include "Diabetes Dictionary," a glossary of terms individuals with diabetes are likely to encounter; "Diabetes Overview;" "Medicines for People with Diabetes;" "Diabetes and Periodontal Disease," a brochure describing the nature of periodontal disease, its relation to diabetes, and proper care of teeth and gums; and "Self-Monitoring of Blood Glucose." FREE. Also available on the web site. Publishes "Diabetes Dateline," a newsletter that summarizes recent research and activities at the National Institute for Diabetes and Digestive and Kidney Diseases (see below). Available in print or electronically, FREE.

NATIONAL INSTITUTE OF DIABETES AND DIGESTIVE AND KIDNEY DISEASES (NIDDKD)
National Institutes of Health
Center Drive, MSC 2560
Building 31, Room 9A-04
Bethesda, MD 20892
(301) 496-3583   www.niddk.nih.gov

Funds basic and clinical research in the causes, prevention, and treatment of diabetes. FREE list of publications. The web site contains fact sheets and patient education materials. Publications available in English and Spanish. FREE

NATIONAL KIDNEY AND UROLOGIC DISEASES INFORMATION CLEARINGHOUSE (NKUDIC)
3 Information Way
Bethesda, MD 20892
(800) 891-5390   (301) 654-4415
FAX (301) 907-8906   www.niddk.nih.gov

Responds to individual requests from the public and professionals about diseases of the kidneys and the urologic system. FREE list of publications. Also available on the web site. Publications available in English and Spanish. FREE

NATIONAL KIDNEY FOUNDATION (NKF)
30 East 33rd Street
New York, NY 10016
(800) 622-9010   FAX (212) 779-0068
www.kidney.org

A professional membership organization that provides professional and public education; produces literature on kidney disease; and promotes kidney transplantation and organ donation.

NEUROPATHY ASSOCIATION
60 East 42nd Street, Suite 942
New York, NY 10165
(800) 247-6968   (212) 692-0662
FAX (212) 692-0668   www.neuropathy.org

This organization serves individuals who experience neuropathy and their family members through the support of research into the causes and treatments of neuropathy, education, and dissemination of information. Membership, FREE, includes newsletter and informational materials.

PUBLICATIONS AND TAPES

THE AMERICAN DIABETES ASSOCIATION COMPLETE GUIDE TO DIABETES
American Diabetes Association
Order Fulfillment
PO Box 930850
Atlanta, GA 31193-0850
(800) 232-6733   FAX (404) 442-9742

This book includes information about type 1 and type 2 diabetes, including how to maintain good blood glucose levels, selecting health care providers, planning an exercise program, and enjoying sex. $23.95

COPING WITH LIMB LOSS
by Ellen Winchell
Avery Publishing Group, Garden City Park, NY

Written by a woman who had a limb amputated, this book provides information about surgery, prosthetics, and rehabilitation as well as practical coping strategies. Out of print

DIABETES AND THE KIDNEYS
American Kidney Fund
6110 Executive Boulevard, Suite 1010
Rockville, MD 20852
(800) 638-8299   (301) 881-3052
FAX (301) 881-0898   www.kidneyfund.org

A booklet that describes how diabetes affects the kidneys' function and measures that may be taken to slow down the course of kidney disease. Single copy, FREE.

DIABETES AND VISION LOSS: SPECIAL CONSIDERATIONS
by Marla Bernbaum
in "Meeting the Needs of People with Vision Loss: A Multidisciplinary Perspective"
Susan L. Greenblatt (ed.)
Resources for Rehabilitation
22 Bonad Road
Winchester, MA 01890
(781) 368-9094   FAX (781) 368-9096
www.rfr.org

This chapter discusses the psychosocial concerns and the special rehabilitation needs of people who have diabetes and vision loss. Print and audiocassette, $24.95.

THE DIABETES CARBOHYDRATE AND FAT GRAM GUIDE
by Lea Ann Holzmeister
American Dietetic Association (ADA)
PO Box 97215
Chicago, IL 60678-7215
(800) 877-1600, ext. 5000   (312) 899-0040, ext. 5000
FAX (312) 899-4899   www.eatright.org

This book lists the carbohydrate and fat content of foods, including packaged foods and foods purchased at fast food restaurants. $14.95

DIABETES: CARING FOR YOUR EMOTIONS AS WELL AS YOUR HEALTH
by Jerry Edelwich and Archie Brodsky
Harper Collins
PO Box 588
Dunmore, PA 18512
(800) 242-7737   www.harpercollins.com

In addition to describing diabetes and its treatment, this book discusses the many effects diabetes has on social and psychological aspects of life. Practical suggestions for adaptation and relationships with medical personnel and family are provided. Information about sexual function, employment, technology, and support groups is also included. $15.00

THE DIABETES HOME VIDEO GUIDE: SKILLS FOR SELF CARE
Joslin Diabetes Center
Publications Department
One Joslin Place
Boston, MA 02215
(800) 344-4501   FAX (508) 285-8382
www.joslin.org

This videotape covers exercise, blood glucose monitoring, nutrition, medications, lifestyle changes, and emotions. Uses people who have diabetes, not actors. 2 hours. Available in English and Spanish. $20.00

DIABETES SELF-MANAGEMENT
PO Box 52890
Boulder, CO 80321
(800) 234-0923   www.diabetes-self-mgmt.com

A bimonthly magazine to help people with diabetes manage their disease. Tips on diet, foot care, medical news, etc. $18.00

DIABETES TYPE 2 & WHAT TO DO
by Virginia Valentine, June Biermann and Barbara Toohey
McGraw Hill, Order Services
PO Box 545
Blacklick, OH 43004
(800) 722-4726   FAX (614) 755-5645
www.mmhe.com

Written in question and answer format, this book addresses the effects of type 2 diabetes including information on diet and nutrition, exercise, emotional aspects, and paying for medical care. Many case examples are presented throughout the book. Includes reading list and Internet resources. Virginia Valentine and June Biermann have diabetes. $16.95

DIABETIC RETINOPATHY: INFORMATION FOR PATIENTS
National Eye Institute (NEI)
Building 31, Room 6A32
2020 Vision Place
Bethesda, MD 20892
(301) 496-5248   www.nei.nih.gov

This booklet discusses the symptoms of diabetic retinopathy, treatment, vitrectomy, and research. Available FREE in LARGE PRINT from NEI and audiocassette ($2.00) from VISION Community Services, 23A Elm Street, Watertown, MA 02472.

THE DIABETIC'S BOOK
by June Biermann and Barbara Toohey
Penguin Putnam, Inc.
(800) 788-6262   www.penguinputnam.com

This book answers basic questions about diabetes, including diet, exercise, management of the disease, emotional responses, and other aspects of daily life. June Biermann has had type 2 diabetes since 1965. $13.95

EXCHANGE LISTS FOR MEAL PLANNING
American Diabetes Association (ADA)
Order Fulfillment
PO Box 930850
Atlanta, GA 31193-0850
(800) 232-6733   FAX (404) 442-9742

This guide lists foods based on carbohydrate, protein, and fat content. $1.75. Discounts available on bulk orders.

THE FIRST YEAR: TYPE 2 DIABETES
by Gretchen Becker
Distributed by Publishers Group West
1700 Fourth Street
Berkeley, CA 94710
(800) 788-3123   FAX (510) 528-3444
www.pgw.com

Written by a woman who has type 2 diabetes, this practical guide includes basic information that people ask about when they are first diagnosed with diabetes. Includes information that helps to cope with the physical, social, and psychological aspects of diabetes. $14.95

GOOD HEALTH WITH DIABETES THROUGH EXERCISE
Joslin Diabetes Center
Publications Department
One Joslin Place
Boston, MA 02215
(800) 344-4501   FAX (508) 285-8382
www.joslin.org

This booklet, written for those who use insulin and those who do not, tells how to get started on an exercise plan, what pitfalls to avoid, and how to integrate exercise with food and medications. $3.45

I HATE TO EXERCISE
American Diabetes Association (ADA)
Order Fulfillment
PO Box 930850
Atlanta, GA 31193-0850
(800) 232-6733   FAX (404) 442-9742

This book promotes the value of 30 minutes of exercise a day to strengthen muscles and the heart and control diabetes. $14.95

THE JOHNS HOPKINS GUIDE TO DIABETES FOR TODAY AND TOMORROW
by Christopher D. Saudek, Richard R. Rubin, and Cynthia Shump
Johns Hopkins University Press
2715 North Charles Street
Baltimore, MD 21218
(800) 537-5487   (410) 516-6900
FAX (410) 516-6998   www.press.jhu.edu/press

Written by a physician, a psychologist, and a nurse who specialize in treating individuals with diabetes, this book provides basic information on diabetes and its treatment, emotional and social aspects of the disease, complications, and sexuality and reproduction. $16.95; LARGE PRINT, $21.50.

LIVING WITH DIABETES $1.75 per copy
LIVING WITH DIABETIC RETINOPATHY $1.75 per copy
Resources for Rehabilitation
22 Bonad Road
Winchester, MA 01890
(781) 368-9094   FAX (781) 368-9096
www.rfr.org

LARGE PRINT (18 point bold type) publications that describe service organizations, publications, and special equipment.

Minimum purchase, 25 copies per title. Discounts available for purchases of 100 or more copies. (See order form on last page of this book.)

LIVING WITH DIABETES: A WINNING FORMULA
Info Vision
102 North Hazel Street
Glenwood, IA 51534
(800) 237-1808   FAX (888) 735-2622
www.infovision.com

This videotape provides information about diet, weight loss, insulin, and self-monitoring of blood glucose and gives recipes. 35 minutes. $25.00

LIVING WITH LOW VISION: A RESOURCE GUIDE FOR PEOPLE WITH SIGHT LOSS
Resources for Rehabilitation
22 Bonad Road
Winchester, MA 01890
(781) 368-9094   FAX (781) 368-9096
www.rfr.org

A LARGE PRINT directory that helps people with sight loss locate the services, products, and publications that they need to keep reading, working, and enjoying life. Information on self-help groups, how to keep reading and working with vision loss, and making everyday living easier. $46.95 (See last page of this book for order form.)

MANAGING DIABETES ON A BUDGET
by Leslie Y. Dawson
American Diabetes Association (ADA)
Order Fulfillment
PO Box 930850
Atlanta, GA 31193-0850
(800) 232-6733   FAX (404) 442-9742

This book provides advice on finding the best buys on supplies
and medications, cooking tips, and general diabetes management. $7.95

MANAGING YOUR DIABETES WITH INSULIN
Joslin Diabetes Center
Publications Department
One Joslin Place
Boston, MA 02215
(800) 344-4501   FAX (508) 285-8382
www.joslin.org

Written for individuals with type 2 diabetes, this booklet provides
information on how to use insulin in their treatment plan. $3.45

A MAN'S GUIDE TO COPING WITH DISABILITY
Resources for Rehabilitation
22 Bonad Road
Winchester, MA 01890
(781) 368-9094   FAX (781) 368-9096
www.rfr.org

This book includes information about men's responses to disability, with a special emphasis on the values men place on
independence, occupational achievement, and physical activity.
Chapter on diabetes includes information about sexual functioning. $44.95. (See last page of this book for order form.)

MAYO CLINIC ON MANAGING DIABETES
by Maria Collazo-Clavell (ed.)
Mayo Clinic Foundation
PO Box 609
Calverton, NY 11933
(800) 291-1128   FAX (631) 369-0615
www.mayo.com

This book provides a basic introduction for newly diagnosed patients and family members. Includes "20 Tasty Recipes for People with Diabetes." $14.95

NATIONAL LIBRARY SERVICE FOR THE BLIND AND PHYSICALLY HANDICAPPED (NLS)
1291 Taylor Street, NW
Washington, DC 20542
(800) 424-8567 (to receive application)
(202) 707-5100   (202) 707-0744 (TTY)
FAX (202) 707-0712   www.loc.gov/nls

Cookbooks written for individuals with diabetes are available from regional library services in each state. Some are available on 4-track audiocassette and some in LARGE PRINT. The NLS refers callers to their regional library.

TAKE CHARGE OF YOUR DIABETES
CDC Division of Diabetes Translation
PO Box 8728
Silver Spring, MD 20910
(877) 232-3422   FAX (301) 562-1050
www.cdc.gov/diabetes

A book written in simple language and printed in LARGE PRINT to help people with diabetes manage their disease. Information on blood sugar, dental, foot, vision, and kidney problems, and nerve damage. Includes forms for keeping records of visits with health care providers and sick days. FREE

A TOUCH OF DIABETES: A STRAIGHTFORWARD GUIDE FOR PEOPLE WHO HAVE TYPE 2, NON-INSULIN DEPENDENT DIABETES

by Lois Jovanovic-Peterson, Charles M. Peterson, and Morton Stone
John Wiley and Sons
Consumer Center
10475 Crosspoint Boulevard
Indianapolis, IN 46256
(877) 762-2974   FAX (800) 597-3299
www.wiley.com

This guide to help people with type 2 diabetes manage their condition includes information about preventing complications and dietary advice. $13.95

THE UNCOMPLICATED GUIDE TO DIABETES COMPLICATIONS

by Marvin E. Levin and Michael A. Pfeifer
American Diabetes Association (ADA)
Order Fulfillment
PO Box 930850
Atlanta, GA 31193-0850
(800) 232-6733   FAX (404) 442-9742

This book covers the major complications that diabetes may cause, including nephropathy, heart disease, stroke, and neuropathy. Special issues such as obesity, pregnancy, and hypoglycemia are also discussed. $18.95

WEIGHT LOSS: A WINNING BATTLE
Joslin Diabetes Center
Publications Department
One Joslin Place
Boston, MA 02215
(800) 344-4501   FAX (508) 285-8382
www.joslin.org

This booklet provides information that helps people control their weight and offers strategies for losing weight. $3.45

WEIGHT MANAGEMENT FOR TYPE II DIABETES: AN ACTION PLAN
by Jackie Labat and Annette Maggi
John Wiley and Sons
Consumer Center
10475 Crosspoint Boulevard
Indianapolis, IN 46256
(877) 762-2974   FAX (800) 597-3299
www.wiley.com

This book provides recommendations for lifestyle changes for weight control and good diabetes management. $15.95

WHAT TO EAT WHEN YOU GET DIABETES
by Carolyn Leontos
John Wiley and Sons
Consumer Center
10475 Crosspoint Boulevard
Indianapolis, IN 46256
(877) 762-2974   FAX (800) 597-3299
www.wiley.com

Written by a dietitian, this book provides guidance to people with type 2 diabetes. Includes information about weight loss, calories, portion size, and carbohydrates. $15.95

A WOMAN'S GUIDE TO COPING WITH DISABILITY
Resources for Rehabilitation
22 Bonad Road
Winchester, MA 01890
(781) 368-9094   **FAX (781) 368-9096**
www.rfr.org

This book addresses the special needs of women with disabilities and chronic conditions, such as social relationships, sexual functioning, pregnancy, childrearing, caregiving, and employment. Written for women in all age categories, the book has chapters on the disabilities that are most prevalent in women or likely to affect the roles and physical functions unique to women including diabetes. $44.95. (See last page of this book for order form.)

SPECIAL EQUIPMENT FOR PEOPLE
WITH VISUAL IMPAIRMENT

Many types of equipment used by individuals with diabetes to monitor and manage their disease are made with LARGE PRINT or speech output. Major distributors of the most commonly used types of equipment are listed below.

ACCU-CHEK VOICEMATE
Roche Diagnostics
9115 Hague Road
Indianapolis, IN 46250
(800) 428-5074   www.accu-chek.com

This talking blood glucose monitor has a feature that identifies insulin vials. Instructions provided in LARGE PRINT and cassette. Available in English and Spanish.

BECTON DICKINSON CONSUMER PRODUCTS
Becton Dickinson & Co.
One Becton Drive
Franklin Lakes, NJ 07417
(888) 232-2737   www.bd.com/diabetes

Sells Magni-Guide with magnification of 2X, that snaps onto Lilly, Nordisk, and Squibb-Novo insulin bottle caps. May be used with 1, .5, and .3 cc syringes.

MEDICOOL, INC.
23520 Telo Avenue, Suite 6
Torrance, CA 90505
(800) 433-2469   (310) 784-1200
www.medicool.com

Sells Count-a-Dose, a device that measures insulin and is used with the Becton Dickinson .5 cc syringe; has tactile marking and audible clicks. Accommodates two insulin vials.

MEDITEC, INC.
3322 South Oneida Way
Denver, CO 80224
(303) 758-6978

Sells the Holdease needle guide and syringe/vial holder and Insulgages, permanent, pre-calibrated for doses ranging from 2 to 85 units. May be marked with print, braille, or raised numbers.

PALCO LABS
8030 Soquel Drive, #104
Santa Cruz, CA 95062
(800) 346-4488   In CA, (831) 476-3151
FAX (831) 476-1114   www.palcolabs.com

Manufactures Insul-eze, which magnifies the syringe calibrations, and Load-Matic, which allows users to set the dosage by touch. Sells the Insulcap, which attaches to an insulin vial, holding both vial and syringe, and guides insertion of syringe.

WHITTIER MEDICAL, INC.
865 Turnpike Street
North Andover, MA 01845
(800) 645-1115   (978) 688-5002

Manufactures the Truhand, a syringe and vial holder with 3x magnifier.

Chapter 6
HEARING LOSS

Government studies indicate that nearly one-third of Americans age 65 or older have hearing impairments. The National Center for Health Statistics (1999) indicates that in 1996, the prevalence rate of hearing impairments in the general population was 83.4 per thousand. Hearing disorders are most common among elders. For those under age 18, the rate was 12.6 per thousand, while for those 75 years or older, the rate was 369.8 per thousand. Projected increases in the older population suggest that the number of people with hearing loss will increase substantially.

Although there are many ways to help elders with hearing loss to continue functioning independently, often people with hearing loss are either embarrassed to seek out help or do not know where to turn. It is not unusual for elders to attribute their hearing loss to the normal process of aging and to think that there is no way to improve their lives. Elders with hearing loss are an underserved population; although they constitute 43% of the total hearing impaired population in the United States, they comprise only 24% of the caseloads of audiologists (Fein: 1983).

Because of the communication problems that hearing loss causes, it often results in a feeling of isolation that in turn may cause severe depression. The inability to communicate with family, friends, and those who provide the daily necessities of life can have an enormous impact on the ability to carry out normal daily activities. Other medical conditions may also be affected when elders with hearing loss have misunderstood directions given by physicians for taking medicine. In extreme cases, such situations may be life-threatening. Inability to hear the telephone ring or to respond to fire alarms also causes dangerous situations.

For some types of hearing loss, surgery may be available to improve hearing. Elders with hearing loss should always receive a complete medical evaluation to determine if medical or surgical intervention will restore hearing; age alone should not rule out medical or surgical intervention.

For those elders with hearing loss that is not amenable to cure by surgery or other medical intervention, there are many ways to improve the standard of living. Most people who experience hearing loss late in life retain some useful hearing. Studies indicate that most elders with hearing loss retain some speech discrimination and the ability to understand the spoken word (Price and Snider: 1983). Elders may learn to improve their ability to communicate by using an increasing variety of assistive devices and by learning special techniques to enhance the utilization of their other senses. Training in the use of hearing aids is essential; experts agree that it is easier for people to learn to use hearing aids and other assistive devices if they are referred for rehabilitation at an early stage in the process of progressive hearing loss. Educating the public about the detection of hearing loss and the wide variety of assistive devices and techniques can be a major factor in assuring that early intervention becomes a reality for more people with hearing loss.

TYPES OF HEARING LOSS

There are a variety of factors that contribute to hearing loss in later life, among them, exposure to loud noise over a long period of time; side effects of drugs prescribed for other medical conditions, including some diuretics commonly prescribed for hypertension; hypertension; and stroke. There are three major types of hearing loss: conductive, sensorineural, and central. Hearing loss that includes both conductive and sensorineural impairments is referred to as mixed hearing loss.

CONDUCTIVE HEARING LOSS is an impairment that prevents sound waves from traveling through the outer or middle ear, on the way to the inner ear. This type of impairment reduces the sound, similar to the reduction of sound resulting from the use of ear plugs. Increased amplification of sound enables the person with this type of hearing loss to understand speech in its normal quality (Price and Snider: 1983). Hearing aids are especially effective with this type of hearing loss.

SENSORINEURAL HEARING LOSS results from damage to the cochlea in the inner ear or to the surrounding hair cells that transmit electrical signals to the nerve fibers and the brain. (For this reason, sometimes elders are told that they have "nerve deafness.") This type of hearing loss is the kind most frequently found in the older population. PRESBYCUSIS, literally the loss of hearing that accompanies old age, is the term that is used to describe hearing loss that occurs in later life and is often used to describe sensorineural hearing loss in elders. Presbycusis is a progressive disorder that may begin quite early in life and affects high pitched sounds most severely. As the condition progresses, middle and lower pitch sounds are also affected (Price and Snider: 1983). Presbycusis usually occurs bilaterally; that is, both ears are affected.

TINNITUS, considered a sensorineural disorder, is the ringing or buzzing sensation that occurs in the ears in the absence of any external sound and frequently accompanies presbycusis. It is estimated that for every 1,000 Americans over age 65, 92.2 experience tinnitus (National Center for Health Statistics: 1991). Although there is rarely a cure for tinnitus, there are ways to alleviate its effects. A tinnitus masker substitutes a more acceptable sound for the sound produced by tinnitus. Tinnitus instruments combine a tinnitus masker with a high frequency emphasis hearing aid. Since each has a separate volume control, the individual can adjust the devices to partially or completely cover up the tinnitus. Because hearing loss often accompanies tinnitus, hearing aids are sometimes effective in alleviating the effects. Other treatments that are frequently prescribed are drugs, surgery, biofeedback, and relaxation techniques.

VESTIBULAR DISORDERS are the result of disease or damage in the inner ear and affect both orientation and balance.

They include vertigo (dizziness); labyrinthitis, an infection of the inner ear, characterized by dizziness, ringing in the ears, and hearing loss; and Meniere's disease, whose symptoms include vertigo, tinnitus, and fluctuating hearing loss. They may be caused by ear infections, blows to the head, whiplash, or stroke-related loss of blood flow to the inner ear or brain. Damage to the inner ear may result in dizziness, nausea, and balance disorders. Hearing loss ranges from mild to total deafness.

CENTRAL HEARING LOSS is less common among elders than conductive or sensorineural hearing loss. Central hearing loss is the result of damage to nerves in the pathway to the brain or in the brain itself. Although sound levels are not affected, speech discrimination is impaired. Central hearing loss is often a secondary result of other medical conditions, including stroke, head injuries, or vascular problems.

The cochlear implant is an inner ear prosthesis used to restore a degree of hearing function in individuals who are profoundly deaf. Electrodes are implanted to bypass the damaged hair cells surrounding the cochlea and stimulate nerve fibers in the ear. After implantation, speech and language professionals devise a rehabilitation plan to help the individual learn to use the implant as effectively as possible. The general criteria for selecting individuals with severe to profound hearing loss to receive the implant include the ineffectiveness of hearing aids in improving auditory recognition, no medical contraindications, and realistic expectations of the results. There is no upper age limit for this surgery, however, individuals must be in good physical health.

The original cochlear implants, using a single channel to stimulate the hair cells, enabled recipients to hear environmental sounds, such as the ring of a telephone or doorbell, traffic noise, and household appliances but not to discriminate speech. Auditory cues such as pitch, when used in conjunction with speech-reading, improved the individual's ability to understand speech. Improved speechreading was the most common result of the earlier generation of cochlear implants (U.S. Department of Health and Human Services: 1988).

Recent advances in technology have expanded the capabilities of cochlear implants. Now they use multiple channels to transmit sound, with the result that many recipients have not only improved speechreading abilities but are also able to recognize speech based solely on auditory recognition. The success of the implant varies with the type of recipient. The most successful are individuals who have developed speech prior to losing their hearing. It is not understood why some individuals are more successful than others in understanding speech following cochlear implantation.

A panel of experts appointed by the National Institutes of Health has recommended that the use of cochlear implants be expanded (NIH Consensus Development Panel on Cochlear Implants in Adults and Children: 1995). The panel recommended that adults with severe hearing impairments who receive only marginal benefits from hearing aids be considered as candidates for cochlear implants.

In 2002, the Food and Drug Administration (FDA) published a notification that a very small percentage of individuals who receive a cochlear implant contract bacterial meningitis. Some individuals with congenital deafness may already be predisposed to contracting this disease, while others who have had otitis media or immunodeficiency status are also at greater risk. The FDA recommends that individuals who are contemplating implantation or who already have implants be vaccinated against the bacteria that cause meningitis.

In 2000, the FDA approved a new device for adults with moderate to severe sensorineural hearing loss. The Vibrant Soundbridge is a surgically implanted hearing device that converts sound into vibrations that are transmitted to the middle ear. Several other implantable middle ear devices are under development.

INDIVIDUALS WITH HEARING LOSS AND VISION LOSS

It is not uncommon for elders to experience problems with both hearing and vision. According to Bagley (1991), professionals in the aging field, health care professionals, and rehabilitation professionals need to make a concerted effort to work together to serve elders with dual sensory impairments. She suggests that service providers look beyond the narrow focus of the particular disability they are trained to work with; that self-help groups be established specifically for groups of people with dual sensory impairments; and that elders have different types of goals than younger people who are involved in rehabilitation. Those who work with elders should advocate to improve the communication and multidisciplinary services available to elders with dual sensory impairments.

Dual sensory impairments have great impact on everyday activities as well as on the ability to use assistive devices. For example, people with both hearing and vision loss often have difficulty manipulating the controls on a hearing aid or replacing the batteries (Bate: 1986). They have difficulty traveling to aural rehabilitation and need to have instructions printed in large type.

PSYCHOLOGICAL ASPECTS OF HEARING LOSS

Depression as a consequence of hearing loss is very common. Studies suggest that people with hearing loss are more likely to be depressed and have low life satisfaction than peers with normal hearing (Glass: 1986). Hearing loss in later life compounds the variety of other losses that are common to elders, such as loss of occupation and associated income, loss of loved ones, and other physical losses. The inability to carry out ordinary conversation and to enjoy social events frequently leads elders with hearing loss to have low self-esteem. Fears of progressive hearing loss and dependency are also common and natural psychological reactions.

Social withdrawal is another psychological reaction that accompanies hearing loss. Because some people find it difficult to accept their hearing loss and seek out appropriate treatment, they try to function as they always did but are unable to do so. Their behavior is often interpreted as mentally inappropriate by family members and friends who are not aware that hearing loss has occurred. In such instances, family members and friends may also withdraw from social encounters. Family and friends withdrawing when communication becomes difficult reinforces the elder's self-devaluation. In extreme cases, elders whose hearing loss has not been diagnosed are inappropriately hospitalized for mental disorders or are placed in nursing homes. One study confirmed the association between cognitive dysfunction and hearing loss among elders, suggesting that clinicians need to be alert to the potential diagnosis of hearing loss in older patients who display symptoms of dementia (Uhlmann et al.: 1989).

Individuals who experience hearing loss later in life often have problems hearing sounds in the higher frequencies. These individuals can hear sounds but are not able to understand the words; their ability to discriminate speech has become impaired. Because consonants are in the higher frequency range than vowels, individuals with impaired speech discrimination may confuse words that have the same roots but different initial consonants. Another problem that is common to people with presbycusis is the inability to understand children, whose voices are high pitched. For elders with hearing loss, this often means an inability to communicate with their grandchildren.

The ability to hear sound but not to understand words and meanings leads some individuals to believe that speakers are mumbling or speaking too softly. This reaction is often accompanied by a denial that hearing loss has occurred. When individuals deny that they have experienced hearing loss, they will be unwilling to seek assistance from professionals who can provide assistive devices or training to improve their communication. Such a situation often causes frustration for family members and friends of the person with hearing loss and may result in increased tensions within the individual's family setting.

When elders accept hearing loss as a "normal" part of the aging process or when they deny that they have a hearing impairment, they are not likely to be successful candidates for rehabilitation. In such cases, it may be helpful to arrange for counseling for both the elder and his or her family members to explain the types of assistance that are available and how they may improve life for all concerned. Another option is to have the elder with hearing loss join a self-help group composed of other elders with hearing loss. (See Chapter 1, "OUR AGING SOCIETY," section on self-help groups). The reluctant elder who learns about others' success and improved lifestyles as a result of aural rehabilitation may decide to accept rehabilitation also.

PROFESSIONAL SERVICE PROVIDERS

The major service providers that work with people with hearing loss are otologists or otolaryngologists, audiologists, and hearing aid dispensers. An examination by a physician is a prerequisite for obtaining a hearing aid.

OTOLOGISTS are physicians who specialize in diseases of the ear. OTOLARYNGOLOGISTS are physicians who specialize in treatment of the ear, nose, and throat. These physicians diagnose and manage diseases that cause hearing problems. For many conditions, medical or surgical treatment results in restoration of hearing. Unfortunately, for most people who experience presbycusis, there is no cure. In order to determine if a condition may be improved with medical or surgical intervention, all individuals with hearing loss should be examined by an otologist or otolaryngologist. Elders should not be discouraged from having a medical evaluation because of the belief that hearing loss is something to be expected with advanced age. In cases where there is no effective medical or surgical treatment to restore lost hearing, the otologist or otolaryngologist should refer the patient to an audiologist or a hearing aid dispenser for evaluation for assistive devices.

AUDIOLOGISTS have special training to administer tests to determine the level of functional hearing; to prescribe hearing aids and other devices; to train patients to use the prescribed devices; to refer patients to other professionals and resources; and to train patients in auditory and visual communication (American Speech-Language-Hearing Association: 1988). Audiologists have either a masters or doctoral degree in audiology and are certified by the American Speech-Language-Hearing Association; in addition, most states license audiologists to practice within the state (Weinstein: 1989). Many audiologists practice in otologists' or otolaryngologists' offices. Others practice in their own private offices, in a hospital or clinic setting, or in a rehabilitation agency.

HEARING AID DISPENSERS sell hearing aids to individuals and are not trained in the diagnosis or treatment of conditions that affect hearing. Some hearing aid dispensers do perform basic audiometric tests. Many, however, sell hearing aids to people who have been referred by audiologists. The Food and Drug Administration (FDA) requires a medical evaluation prior to the fitting of hearing aids. Although individuals may sign a waiver that permits hearing aid dispensers to fit a hearing aid without a medical evaluation, it is wise to be examined by a physician to determine whether the condition that is causing the hearing loss may be amenable to medical intervention and whether the underlying condition is causing other medical problems.

It is essential that primary care physicians and geriatricians screen elders for hearing loss and refer those with hearing impairments to otologists or otolaryngologists and audiologists. Regular screenings may result in earlier rehabilitation and prospects of better results from the rehabilitation process. In addition, primary care physicians should send reports about the patients' general medical condition to otologists or otolaryngologists to ensure that medication and other regimens prescribed by one physician do not have an adverse interaction with those prescribed by the other physician.

A survey of individuals with hearing loss found that all too frequently, patients are not referred for rehabilitation by otologists, otolaryngologists, or audiologists (Glass and Elliott: 1992a). Indeed, the majority of respondents were not aware that vocational rehabilitation services exist (Glass and Elliott: 1992b). Rehabilitation should include prescription of appropriate assistive devices, training in the use of these devices, training in techniques such as lip-reading to enhance communication, and counseling for both the individual with hearing loss and family members.

WHERE TO FIND SERVICES

Many states have special offices to provide services to individuals who are hearing impaired or deaf. These agencies often provide assistive devices, interpreters, vocational counseling, special educational programs, counseling, and advocacy for people with hearing impairments. The specific services and the populations served vary by state. Individuals should contact the state government information operator, the state office serving individuals with disabilities, or the state department of vocational rehabilitation services to determine if an office for people with hearing impairments exists in their state. In addition, state offices of vocational rehabilitation provide services for individuals who are hearing impaired or deaf and are interested in retaining their current positions or receiving training for new careers.

Local agencies providing services to elders with hearing loss include hospitals with otolaryngology departments; private agencies that specialize in services and rehabilitation for individuals who are hearing impaired or deaf; senior citizen centers, which sometimes sell special adaptive equipment; independent living centers; audiologists, otologists, and otolaryngologists in private practice; hearing aid dispensers (listed in the Yellow Pages); universities that have graduate programs for audiologists; and Veterans Administration Medical Centers. Some general rehabilitation facilities provide special rehabilitation for people with hearing impairments.

Public libraries are a good source of directories of local agencies. In addition, some local libraries and museums have special programs for people with hearing problems. An increasing number of performances and social events have special amplification devices available for people with hearing loss (See "ASSISTIVE DEVICES" section below).

ADAPTATIONS FOR ELDERS WITH HEARING LOSS

Any setting where large numbers of elders congregate should be designed to facilitate communications for people with hearing loss. These settings include special housing for elders, senior citizen centers, health care providers' offices, nursing homes, hospitals, rehabilitation centers, and retirement communities. In addition to the environmental suggestions made below, all of these settings should schedule regular hearing screenings conducted by a qualified audiologist to ensure that elders receive early intervention in the event of a hearing loss.

New buildings and those being renovated for use by elders should have good acoustics. For example, curtains and carpets absorb background noise. Amplification systems and assistive listening devices should be installed. Furniture should be placed so that small groups of elders will be close enough to understand each other and are able to see each other clearly.

Elders with hearing loss should consider the wide variety of options available to improve their communication skills. Their own homes should be adapted to facilitate understanding conversations and radio and television programs. In addition, elders should learn about speech-reading, a technique that maximizes visual cues from lip movements and other body gestures, and they should learn to think about the context of the speech. They should always face the speaker during a conversation in order to see these visual cues.

Although some elders may be embarrassed to discuss their hearing loss with friends and relatives, a frank discussion of their disability will help to avoid misinterpretation of conversation that leads to inappropriate responses. Individuals with hearing loss should help others to communicate more effectively by telling them when they have not heard and what the speaker can do to improve the situation, such as speaking louder, facing them, etc. (Trychin: 1995).

Family, friends, and service providers should all learn how to communicate effectively with people with hearing loss. The following tips will save much frustration when holding a conversation with someone who has experienced hearing loss:

· Be certain that the person knows that you are speaking to him or her.

· Always face the person throughout the conversation so that he or she may get visual cues. Be certain that your mouth is visible throughout the conversation even if the person with hearing loss is not an experienced lip reader.

· Be certain that background noises have been eliminated. For example, radios and televisions should not be playing, and water should not be running.

· Speak clearly at a level just slightly above normal, but do not shout.

· If the person does not understand what you are saying, re-phrase the sentence.

· Ask the person if he or she has understood you.

ASSISTIVE DEVICES

The types of devices most appropriate to a given individual depend upon not only the type and severity of hearing loss but also the individual's usual activities. The variety of assistive devices available to help people with hearing loss communicate effectively is constantly expanding. Major organizations such as Self Help for Hard of Hearing People and the American Speech-Language-Hearing Association, (See "ORGANIZATIONS" section below) publish information about a wide range of devices. For those elders who are not able to afford the devices they need, financial assistance is often available through a state agency or through local service organizations. In some states, the agency serving individuals who are hearing impaired or deaf or the vocational rehabilitation agency provides text telephones free on loan or offers them for sale at a discount price. Assistive devices are often available on display at local rehabilitation agencies.

The most common device, the hearing aid, has undergone considerable improvement in recent years, and there are many types and models to choose from. Despite the fact that hearing aids have been available for many years, it has been estimated that only 18% of elders with hearing loss own a hearing aid (Weinstein: 1989). The failure to use hearing aids may be attributed in part to denial of hearing loss, the high cost of some hearing aids, the failure of many medical insurance policies to cover the cost, and improper training in the use of hearing aids. Other disabilities may also interfere with the use of hearing aids. For example, elders with arthritis often have difficulty manipulating small hearing aids, adjusting the controls, and replacing the batteries.

Because hearing aids amplify sound, they amplify background noises as well as conversation. The amplification of background noise is a common reason that some people do not find hearing aids useful. Some hearing aids are designed to screen out certain frequencies and background noises; however, no model is capable of enhancing speech and eliminating background noise perfectly. Advances in hearing aid technology have resulted in a new generation of digitally programmed hearing aids. Audiologists are able to program digital hearing aids so that amplification is specific to the individual's hearing loss at various frequencies. Experts recommend that people with hearing loss purchase hearing aids with a 30 day trial period, so they may be returned or adjusted if not satisfactory.

Assistive listening devices (ALDs) are used in situations where hearing aids are not sufficient. ALDs transmit sound waves directly into the ears of people with hearing loss. They utilize microphones close to the source of the sound, amplifiers, and headsets. Three types of ALDs are infrared, FM, and hard-wired systems. The first two types of systems are useful in group situations and are currently available in settings such as theaters and churches, while the hard-wired system is often useful in the home situation and may be installed inexpensively (Weinstein: 1989). ALDs are sometimes used in conjunction with hearing aids. Individuals with hearing aids with telecoil switches (T switches) use neck loops which transmit sound via magnetic induction signals.

TELETYPEWRITERS (TTYs), also called telecommunication devices for the deaf (TDDs) or text telephone (TTs), transmit printed messages across telephone lines. They utilize computers with screens and keyboards as well as a modem, which serves as the communication device. TTYs may only be used when there is a TTY at the other end of the telephone line. Telephone relay service (TRS) enables parties to communicate by phone when one party does not have a TTY; there is no additional charge for this service. A communications assistant relays the conversation from text to voice and from voice to text. The Americans with Disabilities Act requires that all common carriers provide nation-wide 24-hour TRS service. Telephone companies can provide information about installing a TTY. A TTY operator is available for directory assistance and placing credit card, collect, person-to-person and third party calls. The local telephone directory includes the toll-free number for this service in a section on services for customers with disabilities.

Telephone amplifiers make communication with the outside world available to many individuals with hearing loss. Available in a variety of models, some are easy to use and produce high quality sound, while others are difficult to use and produce inferior sound. Hand-held telephone amplifiers and volume controls attach to phones at home and are useful when traveling. Some states provide telephone amplifiers to qualified users at no charge; the state office that serves individuals who are hearing impaired or deaf should know if the state provides these devices. These devices have become so commonplace that many stores and mail order catalogues that sell phone equipment stock amplifiers as well as TTYs. Federal law in the United States requires that telephones with cords and cordless telephones be compatible with hearing aids.

Visual alerting systems are available to use as smoke or fire detectors and as indicators that the telephone or doorbell is ringing. Dashboard alerting devices may be installed in automobiles to detect emergency vehicle sirens and remind drivers when the turn signal is on. Vibrators are available to substitute for an audible signal from an alarm clock.

Hearing dogs are used in ways that are similar to guide dogs for people with vision impairments. Dogs are trained to lead their owners to the source of sound, such as doorbells, smoke alarms, alarm clocks, and enable people with hearing loss, especially those who live alone, to maintain their independence and security.

Closed captioned television programs, which were relatively rare just a few years ago, are becoming more common, with all major network programs in prime time now closed captioned. Closed captioning provides a print output of the program's speech at the bottom of the television screen. Closed captioned programs are accessible through decoders, which are available through outlets that sell assistive devices for individuals who are hearing impaired or deaf as well as electronics stores such as Radio Shack; they cost about two-hundred dollars or less. The Television Decoder Circuitry Act (P.L. 101-431) mandates that all television sets with screens 13 inches or larger be manufactured with built-in decoders for closed captions. Many videotaped movies available for rental or purchase are also closed captioned. Section 713 of the Telecommunications Act of 1996 (P.L. 104-104) requires that video services be accessible to individuals with hearing impairments via closed captioning.

Interpreted captioning is a system that enables people with hearing loss who are not fluent in sign language or speech-reading to understand the conversation at group meetings (Grant and Walsh: 1990). There are several methods of interpreted captioning, including visual recording, where a volunteer uses large sheets of paper to record the meeting in words, symbols and graphics, and computer assisted real time captioning (CART), where an operator types the dialogue from a meeting into a computer. The computer display may be presented in enlarged form by projection onto a screen or wall; alternatively, large print software may be sufficient to enable members of the group to read the proceedings.

REFERENCES

American Speech-Language-Hearing Association
1988 Position Statement "The Role of Speech-Language Pathologists and Audiologists in Working with Older Persons" ASHA 30(March):80-84
Bagley, Martha
1991 "Older Adults with Vision and Hearing Losses" pp. 71-91 in Susan L. Greenblatt, (ed.) MEETING THE NEEDS OF PEOPLE WITH VISION LOSS: A MULTIDISCIPLINARY PERSPECTIVE Lexington, MA: Resources for Rehabilitation
Bate, Harold L.
1986 "Aural Rehabilitation of the Older Adult" SHHH (May/June):21-23

Food and Drug Administration
2002 "Cochlear Implant Recipients May Be at Greater Risk for Meningitis" FDA PUBLIC HEALTH WEB NOTIFICATION July 24

Fein, D.J.
1983 "Projection of Speech and Hearing Impairments to 2050" ASHA 25(November):31

Glass, Laurel E.
1986 "Rehabilitation for Deaf and Hearing-Impaired Elderly" pp. 218-236 in Stanley J. Brody and George E. Ruff (eds.) AGING AND REHABILITATION New York, NY: Springer

Glass, Laurel E. and Holly H. Elliott
1992a "The Professionals Told Me What It Was, But That's Not Enough" SHHH JOURNAL (January/February):26-28
1992b "The Way Less Traveled Why Not Try Rehabilitation?" SHHH JOURNAL (March/April):28-31

Grant, Nancy C. and Birrell Walsh
1990 "Interpreted Captioning: Facilitating Interactive Discussion Among Hearing Impaired Adults" INTERNATIONAL JOURNAL OF TECHNOLOGY AND AGING 3(Fall/Winter)2:133-144

National Center for Health Statistics
1999 VITAL AND HEALTH STATISTICS, CURRENT ESTIMATES FROM THE NATIONAL HEALTH INTERVIEW SURVEY Series 10, No. 200 DHHS Pub. No. (PHS) 99-1528, Hyattsville, MD: Public Health Service
1991 CURRENT ESTIMATES FROM THE NATIONAL HEALTH INTERVIEW SURVEY, 1990, Series 10, No. 181, DHHS Pub. No. (PHS) 92-1509 Hyattsville, MD: Public Health Service

NIH Consensus Development Panel on Cochlear Implants in Adults and Children
1995 "Cochlear Implants in Adults and Children" JAMA 274:24(December 27):1955-1961

Price, Lloyd L. and Robert M. Snider
1983 "The Geriatric Patient: Ear, Nose and Throat Problems" in William Reichel (ed.) CLINICAL ASPECTS OF AGING Baltimore, MD: Williams and Wilkins

Trychin, Samuel
1995 "It's OUR Hearing Loss" SHHH JOURNAL (May/June) 19-24

Uhlmann, Richard F. et al.
1989 "Relationship of Hearing Impairment to Dementia and Cognitive Dysfunction in Older Adults" JAMA 261(April 7):1916-1919

U.S. Department of Health and Human Services
1988 "Cochlear Implants" NATIONAL INSTITUTES OF HEALTH CONSENSUS DEVELOPMENT CONFERENCE STATEMENT 7(May 4):2

Weinstein, Barbara E.
1989 "Geriatric Hearing Loss: Myths, Realities, Resources for Physicians" GERIATRICS 44(April):42-59

ORGANIZATIONS

ALEXANDER GRAHAM BELL ASSOCIATION FOR THE DEAF
3417 Volta Place, NW
Washington, DC 20007-2778
(800) 432-7543   (202) 337-5220
(202) 337-5221 (TTY)   FAX (202) 337-8314
www.agbell.org

A membership organization that provides services and support for people who are deaf or hearing impaired. Sponsors conferences and workshops. Membership, $50.00; includes "Volta Review," a professional journal and "Volta Voices," a magazine. Members receive a 15% discount on most publications.

AMERICAN SPEECH-LANGUAGE-HEARING ASSOCIATION (ASHA)
10801 Rockville Pike
Rockville, MD 20852
(800) 638-8255   FAX (301) 897-7355
www.asha.org

A professional organization of speech-language pathologists and audiologists. Toll-free HELPLINE offers answers to questions about conditions and services as well as referrals. Provides information on communication problems and a FREE list of certified audiologists and speech therapists for each state. Also available on the web site. Web site also lists self-help groups for individuals with speech and language disorders.

AMERICAN TINNITUS ASSOCIATION
PO Box 5
Portland, OR 97207-0005
(800) 634-8978   (503) 248-9985
FAX (503) 248-0024   www.ata.org

This organization carries out and supports research and education on tinnitus and other ear diseases. Provides audiocassettes of environmental sounds that may provide relief from tinnitus. Membership, $25.00, includes subscription to quarterly magazine, "Tinnitus Today" and informational brochures.

ASSOCIATION OF LATE DEAFENED ADULTS (ALDA)
1131 Lake Street, #204
Oak Park, IL 60301
(877) 348-7537 (V/FAX)   (708) 358-0135 (TTY)
www.alda.org

Sponsors a network of self-help groups for adults throughout the U.S. and Canada who became deaf as adults. Provides information and consultations for professionals and the public. Membership, $20.00; age 62 or older, $15.00; includes newsletter, "ALDA News."

CANINE COMPANIONS FOR INDEPENDENCE
PO Box 446
2965 Dutton Avenue
Santa Rosa, CA 95402
(800) 572-2275, connects to nearest regional center
(866) 224-3647, connects to national headquarters
www.caninecompanions.org

Trains and places hearing dogs with individuals who are hearing impaired or deaf. Services are FREE.

COCHLEAR IMPLANT ASSOCIATION, INC. (CIAI)
5335 Wisconsin Avenue, NW, Suite 440
Washington, DC 20015
(202) 895-2781 (V/TTY)   FAX (202) 895-2782
www.cici.org

A membership organization that provides support and information to individuals prior to and following cochlear implantation. Assists with the formation of local CIAI chapters. Membership, individuals, $25.00; families, $25.00; professionals, $60.00; includes quarterly newsletter, "CONTACT."

DOGS FOR THE DEAF
10175 Wheeler Road
Central Point, OR 97502
(541) 826-9220 (V/TTY)   FAX (541) 826-6696
www.dogsforthedeaf.org

Trains dogs that provide assistance to individuals who are hearing impaired or deaf. These dogs respond to a variety of sounds, such as doorbells, smoke alarms, alarm clocks, etc. One week of training is provided at the recipient's home. All services are FREE.

FEDERAL COMMUNICATIONS COMMISSION (FCC)
445 12th Street, SW
Washington, DC 20554
(888) 225-5322   (888) 835-5322 (TTY)
(202) 418-0190   (202) 418-2555 (TTY)
www.fcc.gov

Responsible for developing regulations for telecommunication issues related to federal laws, including the ADA and the Telecommunications Act of 1996.

GALLAUDET RESEARCH INSTITUTE (GRI)
Gallaudet University
800 Florida Avenue, NE
Washington, DC 20002
(202) 651-5400 (V/TTY)   gri.gallaudet.edu

Conducts research on all aspects of deafness and hearing impairment. Publishes newsletter, "Research at Gallaudet," which reviews research findings. FREE. Some publications are available on the web site.

HEAR NOW
6700 Washington Avenue South
Eden Prairie, MN 55344
(800) 648-4327 (V/TTY)   FAX (952) 828-6946
www.sotheworldmayhear.org

Provides hearing aids to people with limited financial resources. Nonrefundable application processing fee of $39.00 per hearing aid. Recycles donated, used hearing aids.

HELEN KELLER NATIONAL CENTER FOR DEAF-BLIND YOUTHS AND ADULTS (HKNC)
111 Middle Neck Road
Sands Point, NY 11050
(516) 944-8900   (516) 944-8637 (TTY)
FAX (516) 944-7302   www.helenkeller.org/national

Offers evaluation, vocational rehabilitation training, counseling, job preparation, placement, and related services through ten regional offices.

MEDLINEPLUS: HEARING DISORDERS AND DEAFNESS
www.nlm.nih.gov/medlineplus/hearingdisorders.html

This web site provides links to sites for general information about hearing disorders and deafness, symptoms and diagnosis, treatment, prevention/screening, specific conditions/aspects, seniors, organizations, and research. Some information is available in Spanish. Provides links to MEDLINE research articles and related MEDLINEplus pages.

NATIONAL ASSOCIATION OF THE DEAF (NAD)
814 Thayer Avenue
Silver Spring, MD 20910
(301) 587-1788   (301) 587-1789 (TTY)
FAX (301) 587-1791   www.nad.org

A membership organization with state chapters throughout the U.S. Advocates for its members and serves as an information clearinghouse. Special sections for senior citizens, federal employees, and sign language instructors. Holds national and regional conventions. Membership, individuals, $30.00; seniors (over 60), $15.00; includes a newspaper, "The NAD Broadcaster."

NATIONAL INSTITUTE ON DEAFNESS AND OTHER COMMUNICATION DISORDERS (NIDCD)
Building 31, Room 3C35
31 Center Drive, MSC 2320
Bethesda, MD 20892
(301) 496-7243   (301) 402-0252 (TTY)
www.nidcd.nih.gov

Federal agency that funds basic research studies on problems of hearing, balance, voice, language, and speech.

NATIONAL INSTITUTE ON DEAFNESS AND OTHER COMMUNICATION DISORDERS INFORMATION CLEARINGHOUSE
1 Communication Avenue
Bethesda, MD 20892
(800) 241-1044   (800) 241-1055 (TTY)
www.nidcd.nih.gov

Maintains a database of references and responds to requests for information from the public and professionals. Publishes biannual newsletter, "Inside NIDCD Clearinghouse," FREE. FREE publications list.

REHABILITATION RESEARCH & TRAINING CENTER FOR PERSONS WHO ARE HARD OF HEARING OR LATE DEAFENED
California School of Professional Psychology
6160 Cornerstone Court East
San Diego, CA 92121
(858) 623-2777   (800) 432-7619 (TTY)
FAX (858) 642-0266   www.hearinghealth.org

A federally funded research center that focuses on maintaining the employment status and addressing the personal adjustment needs of persons who are hard of hearing or late deafened. Projects include research on pre- and post-surgical adjustment of cochlear implant recipients and mental health issues of persons who are deaf-blind.

SELF HELP FOR HARD OF HEARING PEOPLE (SHHH)
7910 Woodmont Avenue, Suite 1200
Bethesda, MD 20814
(301) 657-2248   (301) 657-2249 (TTY)
FAX (301) 913-9413   www.shhh.org

National membership organization with local and regional chapters. Provides information, support, and individual referrals. Membership, individuals, $25.00; professionals, $50.00; includes subscription to bimonthly magazine, "Hearing Loss: The Journal of Self Help for Hard of Hearing People."

SYMPHONIX DEVICES, INC.
2331 Zanker Road
San Jose, CA 95131
(800) 833-7733   FAX (408) 273-1795
www.symphonix.com

Sells the Vibrant Soundbridge, a surgically implanted hearing device that converts sound into vibrations that are transmitted to the middle ear.

TDI
8630 Fenton Street, Suite 604
Silver Spring, MD 20910
(301) 589-3786   (301) 589-3006 (TTY)
FAX (301) 589-3797   www.tdi-online.org

This organization lobbies for improved telecommunication for individuals who are deaf or hearing impaired. Publishes "National Directory and Resource Guide" annually. Membership, $25.00, includes quarterly newsletter, "GA-SK."

U.S. DEPARTMENT OF VETERANS AFFAIRS (VA)
Prosthetics Division, local VA Medical Centers
(800) 827-1000 (connects with regional office)
www.va.gov

Provides FREE hearing aids to eligible veterans and Tele-Caption decoder for veterans with hearing loss that is service related. In some cases, the VA will pay for cochlear implants.

VESTIBULAR DISORDERS ASSOCIATION
PO Box 4467
Portland, OR 97208-4467
(800) 837-8428   (503) 229-7705
FAX (503) 229-8064   www.vestibular.org

Provides support and information to individuals who experience dizziness, inner-ear balance disorders, vertigo, and related hearing problems. Produces publications and videotapes. Membership, individuals or families, $25.00; professionals, $40.00; includes quarterly newsletter, "On the Level."

PUBLICATIONS AND TAPES

(Publications focusing specifically on assistive devices are listed under "RESOURCES FOR ASSISTIVE DEVICES" below.)

CAPTIONED MEDIA PROGRAM
1447 East Main Street
Spartanburg, SC 29307
(800) 237-6213   (800) 237-6819 (TTY)
FAX (800) 538-5636   www.cfv.org

Offers lending library of videotapes with open captions (no need for decoders). FREE

COCHLEAR IMPLANTS
National Institute on Deafness and Other Communication Disorders Information Clearinghouse
1 Communication Avenue
Washington, DC 20892
(800) 241-1044   (800) 241-1055 (TTY)
FAX (301) 907-8830   www.nidcd.nih.gov

This publication includes information describing how the cochlear implant works, recent articles on the subject, resources, and an annotated bibliography. FREE. Also available on the web site.

COPING WITH HEARING LOSS
by Susan V. Rezen and Carl Hausman
Self Help for Hard of Hearing People (SHHH)
7910 Woodmont Avenue, Suite 1200
Bethesda, MD 20814
(301) 657-2248   (301) 657-2249 (TTY)
FAX (301) 913-9413   www.shhh.org

This book discusses causes of hearing loss, problems experienced by people with hearing loss, solutions for these problems, information about hearing aids, and tips on speechreading. $19.95

COPING WITH HEARING LOSS AND HEARING AIDS
by Debra A. Shimon
Thomson Learning
7625 Empire Drive
Florence, KY 41042
(800) 347-7707   FAX (859) 647-5023
www.thomsonlearning.com

This book discusses the effects of hearing loss, how hearing aids work, and how to buy a hearing aid. $22.95

DEAF OR HARD-OF-HEARING: TIPS FOR WORKING WITH YOUR DOCTOR
American Academy of Family Physicians
11400 Tomahawk Creek Parkway
Leawood, KS 66211-2672
(913) 906-6000   www.aafp.org
familydoctor.org

This fact sheet provides communication tips for individuals who are deaf and use sign language and those who are hard of hearing or deaf and rely on spoken language. FREE. Also available on the web site.

DIRECTORY: INFORMATION RESOURCES FOR HUMAN COM-
MUNICATION DISORDERS
National Institute on Deafness and Other Communication Disor-
ders Information Clearinghouse
1 Communication Avenue
Washington, DC 20892
(800) 241-1044   (800) 241-1055 (TTY)
FAX (301) 907-8830   www.nidcd.nih.gov

This directory describes organizations throughout the country
that deal with communication disorders. FREE. Also available on
the web site.

HEARING LOSS AND OLDER ADULTS
National Institute on Deafness and Other Communication Disorders Information Clearinghouse
1 Communication Avenue
Washington, DC 20892
(800) 241-1044   (800) 241-1055 (TTY)
FAX (301) 907-8830   www.nidcd.nih.gov

This fact sheet describes hearing loss and devices that may be
helpful. Includes a checklist that individuals can use to evaluate
their hearing and a resource list. FREE. Also available on the
web site.

HEAR: SOLUTIONS, SKILLS, AND SOURCES FOR HARD OF
HEARING PEOPLE
by Anne Pope
Self Help for Hard of Hearing People (SHHH)
7910 Woodmont Avenue, Suite 1200
Bethesda, MD 20814
(301) 657-2248   (301) 657-2249 (TTY)
FAX (301) 913-9413   www.shhh.org

This book describes how the ear works and what can go wrong. It also offers practical communication strategies. $19.95

HOW TO SURVIVE HEARING LOSS
by Charlotte Himber
Gallaudet University Press
Chicago Distribution Center
11030 South Langley Avenue
Chicago, IL 60628
(800) 621-2736   (888) 630-9347 (TTY)
FAX (800) 621-8476   gupress.gallaudet.edu

Written by an older woman who has experienced hearing loss, this book describes how she came to terms with her impairment and offers suggestions for coping. $18.95

I SEE WHAT YOU'RE SAYING: LIPREADING PROGRAM
by Mary Kleeman
Alexander Graham Bell Association for the Deaf
3417 Volta Place, NW
Washington, DC 20007
(800) 432-7543   (202) 337-5220
(202) 337-5221 (TTY)   FAX (202) 337-8314
www.agbell.org

This videotape and manual provide instruction in lipreading for adults with hearing loss. Includes many examples in noisy and quiet environments. 54 minutes. $49.95

LEGAL RIGHTS: THE GUIDE FOR DEAF AND HARD OF HEARING PEOPLE
Gallaudet University Press
Chicago Distribution Center
11030 South Langley Avenue
Chicago, IL 60628
(800) 621-2736   (888) 630-9347 (TTY)
FAX (800) 621-8476   gupress.gallaudet.edu

This book discusses federal laws that affect individuals who are hearing impaired or deaf, including the ADA, Social Security, and the Rehabilitation Act. Also includes chapters on employment, telephone and television adaptations, and state programs. $19.95

LIVING WELL WITH HEARING LOSS
by Debbie Huning
John Wiley and Sons
Consumer Center
10475 Crosspoint Boulevard
Indianapolis, IN 46256
(877) 762-2974   FAX (800) 597-3299
www.wiley.com

Written by an audiologist, this book provides practical information about communications, hearing aids, and other issues pertinent to individuals with hearing loss and their families. $12.95

**LIVING WITH HEARING LOSS: THE SOURCEBOOK FOR DEAF-
NESS AND HEARING DISORDERS**
by Carol Turkington and Allen E. Sussman
Facts on File
132 West 31st Street, 17th Floor
New York, NY 10001
(800) 322-8755, extension 4228
FAX (800) 678-3633   www.factsonfile.com

This book provides information about types of hearing loss,
treatment, choosing hearing aids, other assistive devices, and
organizations that serve individuals who are deaf or hearing-
impaired. $16.95

**MISSING WORDS: THE FAMILY HANDBOOK ON ADULT HEARING
LOSS**
by Kay Thomsett and Eve Nickerson
Gallaudet University Press
Chicago Distribution Center
11030 South Langley Avenue
Chicago, IL 60628
(800) 621-2736   (888) 630-9347 (TTY)
FAX (800) 621-8476   gupress.gallaudet.edu

Written by a woman who is deaf and her daughter, this book
describes how families can adjust to a member's hearing loss.
Ms Nickerson, the recipient of a cochlear implant, describes the
barriers she encountered in everyday life after becoming deaf and
her psychological responses as well as her experience adjusting
to this technology. Includes communication methods and information on hearing aids and cochlear implants. $29.95

THE NOISE IN YOUR EARS: FACTS ABOUT TINNITUS
National Institute on Deafness and Other Communication Disorders Information Clearinghouse
1 Communication Avenue
Washington, DC 20892
(800) 241-1044   (800) 241-1055 (TTY)
FAX (301) 907-8830   www.nidcd.nih.gov

This fact sheet describes the causes of tinnitus, possible treatments, and lists resources for further information. Also available in LARGE PRINT. FREE. Also available on the web site.

OLDER ADULTS WITH VISION AND HEARING LOSSES
by Martha Bagley
in "Meeting the Needs of People with Vision Loss: A Multidisciplinary Perspective"
Susan L. Greenblatt (ed.)
Resources for Rehabilitation
22 Bonad Road
Winchester, MA 01890
(781) 368-9094   FAX (781) 368-9096
www.rfr.org

This chapter discusses the special needs of elders with dual sensory losses and how professionals in the fields of health care, rehabilitation, and aging can work together to provide the necessary services. $24.95

TELECOMMUNICATIONS RELAY SERVICES: AN INFORMATIONAL HANDBOOK
Federal Communications Commission (FCC)
445 12th Street, SW
Washington, DC 20554
(888) 225-5322   (888) 835-5322 (TTY)
(202) 418-0190   (202) 418-2555 (TTY)
www.fcc.gov

A booklet that describes how telecommunications relay services work.   Lists telephone numbers to reach communication assistants and to obtain information about this service in each state. FREE. Also available on the web site; click on "Disabilities Issues."

TINNITUS: QUESTIONS AND ANSWERS
by Jack A. Vernon and Barbara Tabachnick Sanders
Allyn & Bacon
160 Gould Street
Needham Heights, MA 02494
(800) 278-3525   www.ablongman.com

This book discusses topics such as the causes of tinnitus, medications, masking devices, tinnitus instruments, support groups, and resources. $28.00

RESOURCES FOR ASSISTIVE DEVICES

Listed below are publications and tapes that provide information about assistive devices and catalogues that specialize in devices for people with hearing loss. Generic catalogues that sell some aids for people with hearing loss are listed in Chapter 3, "MAKING EVERYDAY LIVING SAFER AND EASIER." Catalogues are FREE unless otherwise noted.

ALERTING AND COMMUNICATION DEVICES FOR DEAF AND HARD OF HEARING PEOPLE
Laurent Clerc National Deaf Education Network and Clearinghouse
800 Florida Avenue, NE
Washington, DC 20002
(202) 651-5051 (V/TTY)   FAX (202) 651-5054
clerccenter.gallaudet.edu

A basic guide to the major categories of assistive devices. Available on web site only.

AMERIPHONE
12082 Western Avenue
Garden Grove, CA 92841
(800) 874-3005   (800) 772-2889 (TTY)
(714) 897-0808   FAX (714) 897-4703
www.ameriphone.com

Produces adaptive telephone equipment and television caption decoders.

ASSISTIVE LISTENING SYSTEMS

Architectural and Transportation Barriers Compliance Board (ATBCB)
1331 F Street, NW, Suite 1000
Washington, DC 20004

(800) 872-2253   (800) 993-2822 (TTY)
(202) 272-0080   (202) 272-0082 (TTY)
FAX (202) 272-0081   www.access-board.gov

Describes assistive listening systems. Available in versions for consumers, providers, and installers. FREE. Also available on the web site.

AUTOMOBILITY

DaimlerChrysler Corporation
PO Box 5080
Troy, MI 48007-5080

(800) 255-9877   (800) 922-3826 (TTY)
FAX (810) 597-3501
www.automobility.daimlerchrysler.com

Provides $750 to $1000 reimbursement (on eligible models) on the purchase of alerting devices for people who are deaf or hearing impaired and assistive equipment for vehicles purchased to transport individuals who use wheelchairs.

COMMUNICATION ACCESS FOR PERSONS WITH HEARING LOSS: COMPLIANCE WITH THE AMERICANS WITH DISABILITIES ACT

Mark Ross (ed.)
York Press, Inc.
PO Box 504
Timonium, MD 21094

(800) 962-2763   FAX (410) 560-6751
www.yorkpress.com

This book explains the communications access provisions of the Americans with Disabilities Act and describes communication aids such as FM, infrared, and induction loop systems, amplification devices, interpreters, alerting and signaling devices, and devices to help people with both hearing and vision loss. $37.50

FOOD AND DRUG ADMINISTRATION (FDA)
Office of Consumer Affairs
5600 Fishers Lane
Rockville, MD 20857
(888) 463-6332   (301) 827-4420
FAX (301) 443-9767   www.fda.gov

Distributes publications about hearing aids, which are regulated by the FDA. FREE

GENERAL HEARING INSTRUMENTS, INC.
PO Box 23748
New Orleans, LA 70183-0748
(800) 824-3021   (504) 733-3767
FAX (504) 733-3799   www.generalhearing.com

Sells tinnitus products, such as tinnitus maskers, tinnitus instruments, and low-level noise generators.

GENERAL MOTORS MOBILITY ASSISTANCE CENTER
100 Renaissance Center, PO Box 100
Detroit, MI 48265
(800) 323-9935   (800) 833-9935 (TTY)
www.gm.com/automotive/vehicle_shopping/gm_mobility

This program reimburses customers up to $1000 for vehicle modifications or adaptive driving devices for new or demo vehicles. Includes alerting devices for drivers who are deaf or hearing impaired, such as emergency vehicle siren detectors and enhanced turn signal reminders.

HARRIS COMMUNICATIONS
15155 Technology Drive
Eden Prairie, MN 55344
(800) 825-6758   (800) 825-9187
FAX (952) 906-1099   www.harriscomm.com

Sells products for individuals who are deaf and hard of hearing, such as TTYs, warning devices, clocks and wake-up alarms, assistive listening devices, telephones, and books, videotapes, and CDs. FREE catalogue.

HEARING AIDS
National Institute on Deafness and Other Communication Disorders Information Clearinghouse
1 Communication Avenue
Washington, DC 20892
(800) 241-1044   (800) 241-1055 (TTY)
FAX (301) 907-8830   www.nidcd.nih.gov

This fact sheet discusses types of hearing loss and four basic styles of hearing aids. Provides tips for purchasing hearing aids and how to care for them. FREE. Also available on the web site.

LS & S GROUP INC. CATALOGUE
PO Box 673
Northbrook, IL 60065
(800) 468-4789   (847) 498-9777
www.lssgroup.com

This catalogue includes a variety of devices including clocks, telephones, amplifiers, TTYs, alerting systems, and assistive listening systems. FREE

OVAL WINDOW AUDIO
33 Wildflower Court
Nederland, CO 80466
(303) 447-3607 (V/TTY/FAX)   www.ovalwindowaudio.com

Produces induction assistive listening devices and visual and vibrotactile technology.

PHONIC EAR
3880 Cypress Drive
Petaluma, CA 94954
(800) 227-0735   FAX (707) 781-9145
www.phonicear.com

Produces the Easy Listener, a personal FM amplification system.

SOUND ADVICE ABOUT HEARING AIDS
Bureau of Consumer Protection
Federal Trade Commission (FTC)
600 Pennsylvania Avenue, NW
Washington, DC 20580
(877) 382-4357   (202) 382-4357
(202) 326-2502 (TTY)   FAX (202) 326-2572
www.ftc.gov

This publication makes suggestions for consumers who are considering purchasing a hearing aid; discusses federal and state standards that apply to the sale of hearing aids; and provides information on where to file a complaint, if necessary. FREE

USING A TTY

Architectural and Transportation Barriers Compliance Board (ATBCB)
1331 F Street, NW, Suite 1000
Washington, DC 20004

(800) 872-2253   (800) 993-2822 (TTY)
(202) 272-0080   (202) 272-0082 (TTY)
FAX (202) 272-0081   www.access-board.gov

A brochure with basic information about TTYs (also called TDDs or TTs). FREE

WILLIAMS SOUND CORPORATION

10399 West 70th Street
Eden Prairie, MN 55344
(800) 328-6190   FAX (612) 943-2174
www.williamsound.com

Sells assistive listening devices for personal use and assistive listening systems for group listening.

Chapter 7

OSTEOPOROSIS

Osteoporosis, a condition in which there is too little bone mass, occurs in one out of every four women over 60 (Palmieri: 1988). Although men are also subject to osteoporosis, they generally develop it at a later age than women and comprise about 20% of those with osteoporosis (NIH Osteoporosis and Related Bone Diseases National Resource Center: 2002). Osteoporosis is a major cause of fractures of the spine, hip, and wrist. There are approximately 300,000 hip fractures, 700,000 vertebral fractures, and 250,000 wrist fractures in Americans over age 50 annually. Half of the individuals who experience a hip fracture caused by osteoporosis require some help with daily living, and 15 to 25% enter long term care institutions. The pain and disability associated with osteoporosis have economic consequences that are reflected in medical, nursing home, and social costs. In the United States, the annual costs are estimated at 17 billion dollars (National Osteoporosis Foundation: 2002a).

Although the causes of osteoporosis are not clear, it has been suggested that decreased levels of estrogen and calcium are responsible for weakened bones. Bone strength is also affected by exercise; individuals who exercise regularly lose less bone mass than those who remain sedentary. A study found that post-menopausal women who had previously been sedentary and who carried out supervised weight-lifting exercises twice a week for a year increased their bone mineral density, while a control group who continued in their sedentary lifestyle had a decrease (Nelson et al.: 1994).

The most susceptible individuals are fair-skinned white women who are thin, have small frames, have a family history of osteoporosis, or have had their ovaries removed at an early age (NIH Osteoporosis and Related Bone Diseases National Resource Center: 2002). Other factors associated with the development of osteoporosis are alcohol consumption, cigarette smoking, and the use of certain medications, such as anti-inflammatory drugs.

Loss of height, which occurs when weakened bones in the spine compress, fracture, and collapse, is an early sign of osteoporosis, but the condition is most often confirmed only through the use of x-rays following a fracture. Conventional x-rays do not adequately measure loss of bone mass, but other procedures do, exposing the individual to lower radiation levels. A bone mass measurement, also called a bone mineral density (BMD) test, measures bone density in the spine, hip, heel, hand and/or wrist. Medicare covers bone mass measurement for certain high risk beneficiaries.

Compression fractures of the spine may lead to the development of the "dowager's hump," resulting in loss of height and rounded shoulders. This condition affects the woman's posture and may make her more susceptible to falls. It may also make the individual more prone to breathing problems because the chest cavity is compressed. In individuals with severe osteoporosis, fractures can even be caused by a sneeze, cough, or hug.

To prevent osteoporosis, experts recommend that individuals exercise regularly, stop smoking, use caffeine and alcohol moderately, increase the amount of calcium in their daily diet, and that consider using certain medications (listed below).

In a recent study (2002), Gehlbach and colleagues reported that primary care physicians diagnosed osteoporosis or vertebral fractures in less than 2% of older women and that, of those diagnosed, only a little more than a third were offered appropriate drug therapy. Therefore, it is important that older women initiate conversations with their physicians about their risks of osteoporosis and the need for screening and treatment.

Clinical trials supported by the National Institute on Aging are testing new approaches to maintain or increase bone strength in individuals over age 65. The causes of progressive bone loss in later life are also being studied. A large study of men and their risk factors for fracture and their relationship to bone mass is currently underway at the National Institutes of Health.

TYPES OF OSTEOPOROSIS

Bone tissue is formed, broken down, resorbed, and replaced throughout life in a process called bone remodeling. Cells called osteoclasts dissolve bone tissue, releasing calcium to be used in other parts of the body. The tissue is replaced by osteoblasts, cells that draw calcium and phosphorus from the bloodstream and deposit them on the bones as collagen. In several weeks the collagen hardens to form new bone. According to Lyon and Sutton (1993), the bone remodeling process replaces nearly one-third of an individual's bone tissue in a year.

Bone tissue grows during childhood, adolescence, and early adulthood, peaking between the age of 15 and 30; after age 35, bone loss overtakes bone replacement. PRIMARY OSTEOPOROSIS is seen in both women and men, usually after menopause in women and at a later age in men. Investigators have shown that estrogen has a protective effect on bone which is lost at menopause (National Osteoporosis Foundation: 1989). Bone mass is lost at a more rapid rate after menopause and a woman's risk of fractures increases. After age 70, men lose bone mass at the same rate as women (NIH Osteoporosis and Related Bone Diseases National Resource Center: 2001). SECONDARY OSTEOPOROSIS is the term used to describe bone loss due to a known cause, such as the side effects of certain medications. Glucocorticoids, such as prednisone and cortisone, used to treat asthma, arthritis, and certain types of cancer may lead to loss of bone tissue; anti-seizure medication may affect the calcium supply to the bones; and the use of thyroid hormones may cause bone loss (National Osteoporosis Foundation: 1989). Secondary osteoporosis is more likely to account for bone loss in men and in women before menopause (National Institutes of Health: 2000).

The following factors may help prevent the loss of bone mass and development of osteoporosis:

· GOOD NUTRITION Calcium plays a major role in the development and maintenance of strong bones. The National Academy of Sciences (1997) recommends that all men and women age 65 or over have a daily intake of between 1000 and 1300 milligrams of calcium. Most adults should consume calcium by eating dairy products and other calcium-rich foods such as salmon, broccoli, soybeans, and almonds. Vitamin D, formed in the body after exposure to sunlight, aids the body in absorbing calcium. Individuals who do not receive enough sunlight may need a vitamin supplement. A registered dietitian or nutritionist, physician, or pharmacist can advise individuals which calcium supplements have the best absorption rates, do not interfere with other prescription or over-the-counter medications, and will not lead to excessive calcium intake. Individuals who wish to lower their fat intake and those who have lactose intolerance may substitute skim and low fat milk, yogurt, or lactose-reduced products in order to meet dietary guidelines for calcium intake. Fluoride therapy, which stimulates bone formation and density, is controversial because of undesirable side effects and doubts regarding its effectiveness in preventing hip fractures (Hahn: 1988).

· EXERCISE Walking, jogging, dancing, bicycling, and other forms of weight-bearing exercise are recommended to help decrease bone loss. Activities that involve high loads, such as weight-lifting, are more effective at preventing bone loss than activities that require repetitive motions, such as running or walking. Different forms of exercise benefit different parts of the body; for example, running may result in dense bones in the legs but will not affect the arms or the spine (Brody: 1993). Physical therapists caution individuals with osteoporosis to avoid forward bending during daily activities, which may lead to crush fractures in the spine. Simple exercises which promote good posture and muscle strength will also help prevent injuries.

· HORMONE THERAPY   Although estrogen/progestin hormone therapy has been shown to reduce the number of hip fractures in women, a large clinical study of the effects of this therapy in preventing heart disease, breast and colorectal cancer, and osteoporosis was halted recently due to evidence that the risks outweighed benefits. The Women's Health Initiative study showed a 26% increase in breast cancer, a 41% increase in stroke, and a 29% increase in heart attacks, as well as a doubling of blood clots in legs and lungs, in the women who used hormone therapy (Women's Health Initiative: 2002).   Women are urged to weigh the benefits and their personal risks for these conditions and consider other options for prevention of osteoporosis.

· CALCITONIN, a hormone provided through injection or a nasal spray, has been found to be effective in women with PRIMARY osteoporosis (Avioli: 1992). Although a runny nose is the only side effect reported for the nasal spray form of treatment, allergic reactions, nausea, frequent urination, flushing of the hands and face, and skin reactions are reported side effects of injectable calcitonin (National Osteoporosis Foundation: 2002b).

· FOSAMAX (alendronate sodium), a nonhormonal prescription medication, has been approved by the Food and Drug Administration (FDA) for the prevention and treatment of women after menopause. Since nausea, heartburn, and irritation of the esophagus are possible side effects, it is recommended that a woman take the medication in the morning on an empty stomach, drinking six to eight ounces of water. She should avoid eating, drinking other beverages, or taking other medications, and she should sit or stand upright for at least 30 minutes to an hour after taking Fosamax, to reduce the risk of these side effects. Fosamax should not be taken by individuals with severe kidney disease or low levels of blood calcium. It is also approved for use in treating glucocorticoid-induced osteoporosis in women and in men. In 2000, the FDA approved Fosamax for use in treating primary osteoporosis in men.

· EVISTA (Raloxifene) may be used by postmenopausal women to slow bone loss. It acts like estrogen in increasing bone density but has not been shown to increase risks for breast or endometrial cancer. Women who take Evista may experience hot flashes and leg cramps. Women who have had a history of blood clots in their veins are advised against taking the drug.

· ACTONEL (Risedronate) is approved for use in the prevention and treatment of primary osteoporosis in women and glucocorticoid-induced osteoporosis in both women and men. It has been shown to benefit hip and spine bone mass and decrease spinal fractures. Like Fosamax, it must be taken on an empty stomach, with water, early in the morning, and the individual should remain upright and avoid eating and drinking and taking other medications for at least one half hour.

PSYCHOLOGICAL ASPECTS OF OSTEOPOROSIS

Elders with osteoporosis need to consider changes in their lifestyle to reduce the chance of injury. Such changes may include moving to a home or apartment with only one floor in order to avoid falls on stairs; giving up chores which involve heavy lifting; and learning to use assistive devices in everyday activities. Moving to a new environment, giving up normal routines, and finding new friends require psychological adjustments. Fear of falling often results in activity limitation and staying indoors. The social isolation that results may contribute to loneliness and depression. Elders who find themselves depressed by the multiple changes in their lives may wish to seek counseling from a social worker or psychologist or join a self-help group to learn from others in similar situations.

It is not unusual for elders to become depressed when hospitalized or placed in a long term care facility due to a fracture and to be anxious about their future. Daily living with osteoporosis may require that elders use medication to cope with pain; receive physical therapy to maintain flexibility; and be very cautious in everyday activities. These factors may affect their motivation to participate in a rehabilitation program. The National Osteoporosis Foundation sponsors "Building Strength Together," a network of osteoporosis self-help support groups that provides access to information and emotional support.

PROFESSIONAL SERVICE PROVIDERS

GYNECOLOGISTS often serve as the primary care physicians for women in the age ranges most at risk for osteoporosis. Gynecologists may recommend estrogen replacement therapy for women at menopause, after carefully weighing the benefits and potential risks.

ORTHOPEDIC SURGEONS or PLASTIC SURGEONS may perform surgery to repair or replace bones damaged by fractures caused by osteoporosis. Hip or knee replacement surgery may be recommended.

PHYSIATRISTS, physicians who specialize in rehabilitation medicine, will often first see the individual after a fracture and admission to a rehabilitation program. Physiatrists evaluate the fracture and develop the overall rehabilitation plan. Physiatrists often act as case managers, coordinating medical and rehabilitation services, working with the primary care physician, and arranging for physical therapy, if necessary.

PHYSICAL THERAPISTS design individualized programs to improve posture and strengthen muscles. Physical therapists also teach how to move safely to avoid injury.

OCCUPATIONAL THERAPISTS may perform a home safety assessment, making suggestions for accident prevention such as removing loose electrical cords and throw rugs, installing grab bars, and increasing lighting in stairways, halls, and bathrooms.

REGISTERED DIETITIANS or NUTRITIONISTS recommend dietary measures to ensure that individuals eat the foods that supply important nutrients for the maintenance of their bones.

SOCIAL WORKERS help patients with osteoporosis plan for discharge from a hospital or a rehabilitation center to an environment where they can function independently. This may include discharge to the individual's home with arrangements for home health care; to a relative's home; to a long term care facility; or to congregate housing.

WHERE TO FIND SERVICES

Individuals with osteoporosis will often be hospitalized for corrective surgery when a fracture occurs; when difficult diagnostic procedures are necessary; or for rehabilitation. Individuals may enter a rehabilitation unit within a community hospital or a rehabilitation hospital. Most rehabilitation centers also offer out-patient services.

Elders who have had a fracture may require home health services, including home treatment and maintenance care provided by nurses or home health aides; homemaker services such as meal preparation; Meals on Wheels; chore services such as housecleaning; and adult day activity programs. For some, these services may be needed on a short term basis. They are provided by public and private agencies.

Some of the transportation needs of individuals whose everyday functioning has been affected by osteoporosis may be met through the use of special van services or special parking placards for individuals with disabilities.

ACCIDENT PREVENTION

Individuals who use exercise to maintain strong bones and muscles are less apt to be injured than those who are sedentary. With the following suggestions in mind, elders should perform a safety check of their homes to remove obstacles; they should make other changes to avoid falls and accidents which lead to fractures. Staff members at senior centers and other public areas where elders meet should also be aware of these suggestions:

• Sturdy, low-heeled, soft-soled shoes are safer than high heels with slick soles. Shoes that are too large and slip-on sandals and slippers are also dangerous. Long bathrobes or other full-length garments may result in falls.

• Scatter rugs, loose telephone and electric cords, and clutter should be removed. Nonskid mats should be used in bathtubs and showers, and grab bars should be installed.

• Night-lights should be used in bathrooms and halls, and bright bulbs should be used in stairs and halls.

• Handrails should be installed in stairways, and treads or carpeting used on stairs should be firmly fastened down.

• Caution should be used on wet, icy, uneven, or broken pavement. Curbs, slick floors, tile floors, and oil leaks present hazards to elders with osteoporosis.

• Elders should ask their physicians about side effects of medications, such as dizziness, balance problems, or light-headedness. The use of alcohol may also affect balance and reflexes.

• Elders should have their vision and hearing checked regularly. Inadequate refraction for eyeglasses or the build-up of ear wax may cause balance problems.

• Elders should consult with a physical therapist for suggestions to help reduce their risk for fractures. Proper sitting and standing positions, correct pulling and pushing techniques, and reducing stress on the back and joints when sleeping or resting will enable elders to live more comfortably with osteoporosis.

REFERENCES

Avioli, Louis V.
1992 "Osteoporosis Syndromes: Patient Selection for Calcitonin Therapy" GERIATRICS 47(April)4:58-67

Brody, Jane E.
1993 "Exercise Helps Protect Bones, but Not Alone" INTERNATIONAL HERALD TRIBUNE July 15

Gehlbach, S.H., M. Fournier, and C. Bigelow
2002 "Recognition of Osteoporosis by Primary Care Physicians" AMERICAN JOURNAL OF PUBLIC HEALTH 92:2(February):271-273

Hahn, Bevra H.
1988 "Osteoporosis: Diagnosis and Management" BULLETIN ON THE RHEUMATIC DISEASES 38:1-9 Atlanta, GA: Arthritis Foundation

Lyon, Wanda S. and Cynthia E. Sutton
1993 OSTEOPOROSIS: HOW TO MAKE YOUR BONES LAST A LIFETIME Orlando, FL: Tribune Publishing

National Academy of Sciences
1997 DIETARY REFERENCE INTAKES FOR CALCIUM, PHOSPHORUS, MAGNESIUM, VITAMIN D, AND FLUORIDE Washington, DC: National Academy Press

National Institutes of Health
2000 OSTEOPOROSIS PREVENTION, DIAGNOSIS, AND THERAPY NIH CONSENSUS STATEMENT ONLINE 2000 March 27-29; [2002:8:1]; 17(1):1-36

National Institutes of Health Osteoporosis and Related Bone Diseases National Resource Center
2002 FAST FACTS ON OSTEOPOROSIS Washington, DC: NIH Osteoporosis and Related Bone Diseases-National Resource Center

2001   OSTEOPOROSIS IN MEN Washington, DC: NIH
       Osteoporosis and Related Bone Diseases-National
       Resource Center
National Osteoporosis Foundation
2002a PREVALENCE OF LOW BONE MASS AND OSTEOPOROSIS
       AFFECTS SIGNIFICANT PERCENTAGE OF MEN AND
       WOMEN IN U.S. 50 AND OLDER Washington, DC: National
       Osteoporosis Foundation
2002b MEDICATIONS AND OSTEOPOROSIS Washington, DC:
       National Osteoporosis Foundation
1989   BONING UP ON OSTEOPOROSIS Washington, DC: National
       Osteoporosis Foundation
Nelson, M. et al.
1994   "Effects of High Intensity Strength On Multiple Risk Factors
       for Osteoporotic Fractures: A Randomized Controlled Trial"
       JAMA 272(Dec 28):1909-14
Palmieri, Genaro M.A.
1988   "Prevention and Treatment of Osteoporosis" CLINICAL
       REPORT ON AGING 2:19-20 New York, NY: American Geria-
       trics Society
Women's Health Initiative
2002   "Risks and Benefits of Estrogen Plus Progestin in Healthy
       Postmenopausal Women" JAMA 288:3(July 17):321-333

ORGANIZATIONS

AMERICAN ACADEMY OF ORTHOPAEDIC SURGEONS
6300 North River Road
Rosemont, IL 60018
(800) 346-2267   (847) 823-7186
FAX (847) 823-8125   orthoinfo.aaos.org

A professional organization for orthopaedic surgeons and allied health professionals. Web site offers a "Find a Surgeon" link. Click on "Spine" for fact sheets. A quarterly e-mail newsletter, "Your Orthopaedic Connection," is available upon request.

AMERICAN CHRONIC PAIN ASSOCIATION (ACPA)
PO Box 850
Rocklin, CA 95677
(916) 632-0922   FAX (916) 632-3208
www.theacpa.org

Organizes groups throughout the U.S. to provide support and activities for people who experience chronic pain. $30.00 first year, $15.00 thereafter; includes quarterly newsletter, "ACPA Chronicle."

AMERICAN DIETETIC ASSOCIATION (ADA)
216 West Jackson Boulevard
Chicago, IL 60606
(800) 366-1655   (312) 899-0040
FAX (312) 899-1758   www.eatright.org

Consumers may receive a referral to a registered dietitian or receive information about nutrition on the telephone or on the web site. Available in English and Spanish.

AMERICAN PAIN FOUNDATION (APF)
201 North Charles Street, Suite 710
Baltimore, MD 2120
(888) 615-7246   FAX (410) 385-1832
www.painfoundation.org

This organization provides educational materials and advocates on behalf of people who are experiencing pain. Promotes research and advocates to remove barriers to treatment for pain. Distributes patient educational materials, FREE, and has information about the causes of pain and treatment as well as links to related sites on its web site.

BUILDING STRENGTH TOGETHER
National Osteoporosis Foundation (NOF)
1232 22nd Street, NW
Washington, DC 20037
(202) 223-2226   www.nof.org

The Foundation provides a support group manual, educational materials, referrals, and technical support to individuals who start osteoporosis support groups. FREE

MEDLINEPLUS: OSTEOPOROSIS
www.nlm.nih.gov/medlineplus/osteoporosis.html

This web site provides links to sites for general information about osteoporosis, symptoms and diagnosis, treatment, prevention/screening, specific conditions/aspects, clinical trials, nutrition, research, and organizations. Includes an interactive tutorial. Some information is available in Spanish. Provides links to MEDLINE research articles and related MEDLINEplus pages.

NATIONAL INSTITUTE OF ARTHRITIS AND MUSCULOSKELETAL AND SKIN DISEASES (NIAMS)
Building 31, Room 4C05
31 Center Drive, MSC 2350
Bethesda, MD 20892
(301) 496-8190   FAX (301) 480-2814
www.niams.nih.gov

Sponsors specialized research centers in rheumatoid arthritis, osteoarthritis, and osteoporosis. These centers conduct basic and clinical research; provide professional, public, and patient education; and are involved in community activities. Also supports individual clinical and basic research.

NATIONAL INSTITUTE OF ARTHRITIS AND MUSCULOSKELETAL AND SKIN DISEASES INFORMATION CLEARINGHOUSE
1 AMS Circle
Bethesda, MD 20892
(877) 226-4267   (301) 495-4484
(301) 565-2966 (TTY)   FAX (301) 718-6366
www.niams.nih.gov

Distributes information, bibliographies, and fact sheets about osteoporosis. FREE. Also available on the web site.

NATIONAL INSTITUTES OF HEALTH OSTEOPOROSIS AND RELATED BONE DISEASES NATIONAL RESOURCE CENTER
1232 22nd Street, NW
Washington, DC 20037
(800) 624-2663   (202) 223-0344
FAX (202) 223-2237   www.osteo.org

Provides public and professional education materials on metabolic bone diseases including osteoporosis. Makes referrals to physicians and support groups.   Publishes quarterly newsletter, "NIH ORBD-NRC NEWS." FREE

NATIONAL OSTEOPOROSIS FOUNDATION (NOF)
1232 22nd Street, NW
Washington, DC 20037
(202) 223-2226   www.nof.org

Provides public and professional education materials and supports research.   FREE.   Membership, $15.00, includes quarterly newsletter, THE OSTEOPOROSIS REPORT, and discounts on educational materials. Web site offers links to an online video library of topics such as understanding osteoporosis, risk factors, bone density testing, and treatment.

SPINE-HEALTH.COM
1840 Oak Avenue, Suite 112
Evanston, IL 60201
www.spine-health.com

This web site provides information on coping with chronic back pain, treatment, pain management, and rehabilitation. Also offers a physician directory on the web site.

PUBLICATIONS

AFTER THE VERTEBRAL FRACTURE
NIH Osteoporosis and Related Bone Diseases National Resource
Center (ORBD)
1232 22nd Street, NW
Washington, DC 20037
(800) 624-2663   (202) 223-0344
(202) 466-4315 (TTY)   FAX (202) 223-2237
www.osteo.org

This fact sheet discusses vertebral fractures, treatment, and rehabilitation. FREE

BONING UP ON OSTEOPOROSIS
National Osteoporosis Foundation (NOF)
1232 22nd Street, NW
Washington, DC 20037
(202) 223-2226   FAX (202) 223-2237
www.nof.org

This handbook provides information on the causes, diagnosis, prevention, and treatment of osteoporosis. Members, FREE; nonmembers, $3.00.

FACTS ABOUT OSTEOPOROSIS, ARTHRITIS, AND OSTEOARTHRITIS
National Osteoporosis Foundation (NOF)
1232 22nd Street, NW
Washington, DC 20037
(202) 223-2226   FAX (202) 223-2237
www.nof.org

This booklet discusses the difference between osteoporosis and arthritis and how treatment for arthritis may affect the development of osteoporosis. FREE

FALLS AND RELATED FRACTURES
National Osteoporosis Foundation (NOF)
1232 22nd Street, NW
Washington, DC 20037
(202) 223-2226   FAX (202) 223-2237
www.nof.org

This brochure describes the relationship between osteoporosis and falls and fractures. Suggests prevention strategies and balance exercises. FREE

HOME SAFETY CHECKLIST FOR OLDER CONSUMERS
U.S. Consumer Product Safety Commission
Washington, DC 20207
(800) 638-2772   www.cpsc.gov

Provides information on simple, inexpensive repairs and safety recommendations. Available in English and Spanish. FREE. Also available on the web site.

LIVING WITH OSTEOPOROSIS
National Osteoporosis Foundation (NOF)
1232 22nd Street, NW
Washington, DC 20037
(202) 223-2226   FAX (202) 223-2237
www.nof.org

This booklet provides tips for everyday living with osteoporosis. Includes recommendations for preventing falls and making every room in the home fall-safe. FREE

MEDICATIONS AND BONE LOSS
National Osteoporosis Foundation (NOF)
1232 22nd Street, NW
Washington, DC 20037
(202) 223-2226   FAX (202) 223-2237
www.nof.org

This booklet discusses how medications such as steroids, taken for other medical conditions, may increase the risk of developing osteoporosis. FREE

MEN WITH OSTEOPOROSIS: IN THEIR OWN WORDS
National Osteoporosis Foundation (NOF)
1232 22nd Street, NW
Washington, DC 20037
(202) 223-2226   FAX (202) 223-2237
www.nof.org

This booklet describes the prevention, diagnosis, and treatment of osteoporosis in men. FREE

OSTEOPOROSIS
Arthritis Foundation
PO Box 7669
Atlanta, GA 30357-0669
(800) 283-7800   (404) 872-7100
FAX (404) 872-0457   www.arthritis.org

This booklet provides information about causes, symptoms, diagnosis, and treatment of osteoporosis. Includes home safety check list. $1.00

OSTEOPOROSIS AND ARTHRITIS: TWO COMMON BUT DIFFERENT CONDITIONS
NIH Osteoporosis and Related Bone Diseases National Resource Center (ORBD)
1232 22nd Street, NW
Washington, DC 20037
(800) 624-2663   (202) 223-0344
(202) 466-4315 (TTY)   FAX (202) 223-2237
www.osteo.org

This brochure provides an overview of the risk factors, physical effects, treatment options, and pain management strategies associated with osteoporosis, osteoarthritis, and rheumatoid arthritis. FREE. Also available on the web site.

OSTEOPOROSIS: A WOMAN'S GUIDE
National Osteoporosis Foundation (NOF)
1232 22nd Street, NW
Washington, DC 20037
(202) 223-2226   FAX (202) 223-2237
www.nof.org

This brochure describes how women can assess their risk for the condition and prevent or slow its progress. Available in standard print and LARGE PRINT. FREE

PREVENTING OSTEOPOROSIS
American College of Obstetricians and Gynecologists
409 12th Street, SW, PO Box 96920
Washington, DC 20024
(202) 638-5577   FAX (202) 484-1595
Resource Center: (202) 863-2518
www.acog.org

This brochure describes the condition, risk factors, and prevention. Discusses hormone replacement therapy and includes a chart of foods containing calcium. FREE

STAND UP TO OSTEOPOROSIS
National Osteoporosis Foundation (NOF)
1232 22nd Street, NW
Washington, DC 20037
(202) 223-2226   FAX (202) 223-2237
www.nof.org

This booklet describes the diagnosis, prevention, and treatment of osteoporosis. FREE

2002 DRUG GUIDE
Arthritis Foundation
PO Box 7669
Atlanta, GA 30357-0669
(800) 283-7800   (404) 872-7100
FAX (404) 872-0457   www.arthritis.org

This guide, published annually, reviews the drugs used in treating osteoporosis as well as arthritis and other related conditions. Includes a "Drug and Dosage Diary." FREE

PARKINSON'S DISEASE

:inson's disease, a degenerative, progressive disease, is characterized by the loss of nerve cells in a portion of the brain called the substantia nigra. These cells produce dopamine, a chemical that transmits nerve signals which control movement. Symptoms of Parkinson's disease include tremor, rigidity or muscular stiffness, bradykinesia or slow body movement, and balance problems. Tremor may affect one limb or one side of the body at first, but it often spreads to the other side of the body as the disease progresses. A positive diagnosis for Parkinson's disease cannot be made until diagnostic tests such as an electroencephalogram (EEG) or magnetic resonance imaging (MRI) have ruled out other conditions with similar symptoms. Although there is no cure for Parkinson's disease, medication and special exercises improve functioning in many individuals.

About 50,000 individuals are diagnosed with Parkinson's disease each year; it affects more than 500,000 individuals in the United States (National Institute of Neurological Disorders and Stroke: 2001). Although Parkinson's disease occurs primarily in elders, about 5% of all individuals with Parkinson's disease develop symptoms before the age of 40 (Stern and Mackenzie: 1991). While most individuals experience idiopathic Parkinson's disease (the cause of the disease is unknown), some individuals experience drug-induced Parkinson's as a result of medication prescribed to treat mental disorders. For these individuals, the Parkinson's symptoms are reversed when medication is discontinued. In a small proportion of individuals, symptoms of Parkinson's disease may be the result of brain tumors, carbon monoxide poison or other toxins, or trauma due to repeated blows to the head.

In recent years, however, research has focused on genetic aspects of the disease, raising hopes that new treatments and a possible cure may be found (Duvoisin and Sage: 1996). In 1997,

232

scientists at the National Institutes of Health reported discovery of a gene defect responsible for a form of early onset Parkinson's disease. Despite the fact that this gene defect has been implicated in only a small number of cases, this discovery will serve as a basis for future research. Several recent studies have found genetic factors that are thought to influence an individual's susceptibility to late-onset Parkinson's disease in combination with environmental factors.

Some observers believe that Parkinson's disease is present in a latent phase before any symptoms appear (Koller: 1992). Symptoms may be intermittent at first, or individuals may experience fatigue, aches and pains, irritability, and lack of energy before the classic symptoms of Parkinson's disease appear.

The loss of control of body movements interferes with even simple everyday activities. For example, tremor affects holding a book, a newspaper, and eating utensils. Rigidity causes fine motor problems, which cause difficulty in activities such as buttoning a shirt or tying shoes. Bradykinesia interferes with rising from a chair, putting on a coat, blinking, swallowing, and even facial expression. "Freezing" or akinesia is a sudden inability to move while walking. In addition, the inability to control body movement often causes individuals to walk in a stooped position, affecting balance and causing falls. Falls, in turn, may lead to other complications such as hip fractures or head injuries. A loss of independence often ensues following these injuries. (See Chapter 3, "MAKING EVERYDAY LIVING SAFER AND EASIER," section on Falls and Safety.)

Other symptoms include drooling and difficulties swallowing; a sluggish gastrointestinal system; and frequent urges to void the bladder, even when it is not full. The gait of individuals with Parkinson's disease is characterized by small, shuffling steps. Low blood pressure when standing is also symptomatic of Parkinson's disease. Some individuals experience visual problems because poor muscle coordination results in irregular eye movements; at times they may be unable to blink, due to "freezing."

Although most people with Parkinson's disease retain their mental faculties, in the later stages of the disease some individuals become confused or forgetful and exhibit other signs of dementia.

Medical treatment for Parkinson's disease begins when individuals experience functional losses that interfere with everyday life. Sinemet, the most commonly used drug for Parkinson's disease, is a combination of levodopa (sometimes referred to as L-dopa) and carbidopa. Levodopa is the ingredient that controls the symptoms, while carbidopa enhances its efficacy and eliminates some of its side effects. Long term usage of levodopa often results in decreased benefits and greater side effects. In order to maximize its efficacy, the lowest dose possible is prescribed at the outset.

Other drugs, called dopamine agonists because they mimic the action of dopamine, may be used prior to levodopa or in combination with it. Bromocriptine, pergolide, pramipexole and ropinirole are used in treating both early and advanced Parkinson's disease. Common side effects, such as low blood pressure, dizziness, and lethargy, may be reduced by introducing and increasing agonist dosage very slowly.

A drug called selegiline (Eldepryl) is prescribed to retard the breakdown of dopamine. It may be used alone or in combination with Sinemet. Physicians may adjust medications at various stages of the disease to maximize relief of symptoms and minimize side effects. For example, individuals who experience a "wearing off" of drug therapy may be advised to take smaller doses more frequently.

In January, 1998, the Food and Drug Administration (FDA) approved a drug called tolcapone (Tasmar), a COMT inhibitor. COMT inhibitors block an enzyme that breaks down levodopa before it reaches the brain. Tasmar is taken along with levodopa to prolong the reduction of symptoms and improve motor function. However, in November, 1998, the FDA and the manufacturer issued a warning regarding the use of Tasmar, due to reports of three deaths from liver failure. Package labels now recommend increased liver monitoring (every two weeks); discontinuance after an initial three week treatment, if substantial symptom relief is not observed; and the use of an informed consent document to insure that patients understand the risks of taking the drug. Entacapone (Comtan), another COMT inhibitor approved by the FDA in 1999, does not cause the liver problems of Tasmar and may be tried first. There is disagreement among neurologists over the best time to start COMT inhibitors (Movement Disorder Society: 2002). Some physicians believe that taking these drugs early in the disease's course results in better motor control and reduces the risk of developing motor complications. Others believe that early COMT usage leads to earlier motor complications.

In 2002, the FDA approved the expanded use of Activa Parkinson's Control Therapy, a deep brain stimulator that uses an electrode implanted in the brain, connected to a battery powered programmable electronic stimulator that is implanted in the abdomen or chest (Food and Drug Administration: 2002). The individual holds a magnet over the stimulator in order to activate it. The electrical signals transmitted by the device interfere with nerve cells that cause tremors. The procedure was initially approved in 1997 for use in one side of the brain only; now it may be used in both sides, but requires two separate systems. Despite improvements in motor skills, study participants experienced side effects such as pain and infection, bleeding in the brain, and weakness.

A study is now underway of patients taking Coenzyme Q10, available as a dietary supplement, to evaluate whether it can slow the progression of Parkinson's disease symptoms (National Parkinson Foundation: 1998).

Individuals who have been on anti-Parkinson medications for an extended period of time may also experience an "on-off" reaction. This reaction involves sudden changes from dyskinesia, or uncontrolled movements, to akinesia, or the lack of movement. The "on-off" reaction may occur frequently throughout the course of a day, although it is not possible to predict when the "on-off" reaction will occur. Adjustments in medication dosage or schedule may reduce the "on-off" reaction.

Other medical conditions must also be considered when treating Parkinson's disease. Some medications for Parkinson's disease may interfere with the treatment for other conditions, such as narrow angle glaucoma and heart disease. On the other hand, some blood pressure medications may exacerbate the symptoms of Parkinson's disease. Anti-depressant, anti-psychotic, and anti-vomiting drugs should not be taken by individuals with Parkinson's disease (Lieberman et al.: 1993). The physician and patient must work together to find the best treatment to maintain everyday function.

Exercises may improve balance and flexibility, relieve tight muscles and poor posture, facilitate getting out of a bed or chair, reduce stress, and maintain a feeling of well-being. Physical therapists are able to assess the individual's condition and prescribe an exercise regimen. Individuals with speech problems may be encouraged to practice deep breathing, do facial exercises, and to sing or read out loud, using a tape recorder to note any changes in pitch or inflection.

The National Institute on Neurological Disorders and Stroke (NINDS) is currently conducting research on improved drugs, new delivery systems such as portable infusion pumps, and brain cell transplantation experiments with animals. The development of positron emission tomography (PET scan) allows observation of chemical changes in the brain as a person carries out a routine activity, enabling comparison of brain activities in individuals with Parkinson's disease to brain activities of individuals who do not have Parkinson's disease.

Pallidotomy is a surgical procedure in which the abnormal brain cells thought to be responsible for Parkinson's disease are destroyed. Recent studies using relatively small samples of patients suggest that movement disorders caused by Parkinson's, such as bradykinesia, rigidity, and tremor, have decreased following pallidotomy and that the improvements remained for the year of follow-up. Patients were required to continue their medication after surgery (Dogali et al.: 1995).

Several studies have investigated the benefits of transplanting human fetal tissue containing dopamine cells into the brains of patients with Parkinson's disease. Although these studies involved small numbers of patients, the results suggest that patients who received these transplants experienced moderate improvement in functioning, especially in the area of motor tasks, and were able to reduce their level of medication (Freed et al.: 1992; Spencer et al.: 1992). Gene therapy and stem cell implants are currently being investigated as well.

PSYCHOLOGICAL ASPECTS OF PARKINSON'S DISEASE

Individuals with Parkinson's disease often experience depression, although it is often overlooked by health care providers; whether the cause of this depression is organic or whether it is a result of living with a chronic and progressive disease is unknown. Living with a progressive disease may cause anxiety and fear, as the future is fraught with uncertainty. An international study of patients with Parkinson's disease, caregivers, and clinicians found that half of the patients were depressed despite the fact that few subjects reported that they experienced depression (Phillips: 1999). Both psychological counseling and participation in self-help groups may help to alleviate depression and anxiety. By sharing practical suggestions with members of a self-help group, individuals with Parkinson's disease may focus their energy on activities that relieve their symptoms and build self-esteem. Anti-depressant medications may relieve symptoms. There have been conflicting opinions regarding the prescription of some common anti-depressants for individuals who are also taking selegiline (Eldepryl). In some instances, the symptoms of Parkinson's disease may cause individuals to appear depressed when they are not. The disease affects speech, making it soft, monotonous, and often rapid, with words and syllables running together; facial expression, which often appears emotionless; and posture, which is often stooped.

Family relations are often strained as a result of Parkinson's disease. Family members may become impatient with the individual who walks and eats slowly. Sleep disturbances, common in individuals with Parkinson's disease, may also affect the spouse's sleep. Medication may affect sexual activity, causing impotence, vaginal dryness, or persistent and painful erections. A change of medication; treatment with sildenafil citrate (Viagra) for erectile dysfunction; the use of a commercial, water soluble lubricant; or planning sexual activity after the first medication of the day takes effect are possible solutions (Lieberman et al.: 1993). Often role reversals are necessary, with the healthy partner taking on new responsibilities formerly carried out by the partner with Parkinson's disease. Medical expenses may require a spouse to acquire an additional job, while at the same time caregiving duties have increased. In some instances, the family may be overprotective, not allowing the individual with Parkinson's disease to do as much as possible. The individual often feels helpless, the family overburdened.

PROFESSIONAL SERVICE PROVIDERS

INTERNISTS or FAMILY PHYSICIANS coordinate the individual's overall care and make referrals to specialists when specific symptoms interfere with normal function. NEUROLOGISTS are physicians who diagnose and treat conditions involving the brain and nervous system. PHYSIATRISTS, physicians who specialize in rehabilitation medicine, assess the individual's symptoms and functional limitations and make referrals for physical, occupational, and speech therapy.

PHYSICAL THERAPISTS develop a daily exercise program to enable the individual to maintain posture, remain mobile, and conserve energy. Good muscle tone and agility maximize the individual's physical abilities and self-confidence.

OCCUPATIONAL THERAPISTS assess the individual's functioning in activities of everyday living in his or her home; recommend and provide training in the use of adaptive equipment; and work with families to encourage independence.

SPEECH THERAPISTS or SPEECH PATHOLOGISTS help the individual with speech and swallowing problems to maintain the best possible speech and communication. Consultations with DIETITIANS who suggest dietary modifications to improve chewing or swallowing may also be helpful.

WHERE TO FIND SERVICES

Physical therapy, speech therapy, and occupational therapy are offered by professionals who work in hospitals, private practice, and home health agencies. Local chapters of national voluntary organizations offer counseling, self-help groups, public and professional education, publications, and discount drug programs. Many Parkinson's disease self-help programs offer exercise, speech therapy, and stress reduction groups to their participants. Self-help groups may also provide support to the spouse/caregiver, family members, and others.

Adult day care centers located in hospitals, senior centers, and other private agencies, provide respite care for elders who might otherwise require institutionalization. This service is often free to elders who meet income guidelines, or fees may be on a sliding scale.

ASSISTIVE DEVICES

There are many assistive devices which enable individuals with Parkinson's disease to perform activities of daily living.

Some devices are readily available in medical supply stores and through mail order catalogues, while others require a prescription from a health care professional (See Chapter 3, "MAKING EVERYDAY LIVING SAFER AND EASIER").

A reading stand will hold material steady for an individual with tremor. Utensils with built-up handles and plate guards make eating easier; weighted pens and various grips assist in writing. Clothing with velcro fasteners, elastic shoelaces, buttoning aids, and a long handle shoehorn will help the individual with rigidity to dress more easily. Slowness of movement may be reduced with the use of ambulation aids such as a cane, quad cane (a support cane with a four legged base), or walker. Grab bars in the tub or shower and the use of a nonslip bathmat, shower chair, and raised toilet seat facilitate bathing. Some individuals with Parkinson's disease find that satin sheets, a firm mattress, and siderails make it easier to get out of bed.

Speech amplification devices, such as a portable microphone, are useful for those who have difficulty speaking at normal volume. Speaker phones, telephone operator headsets and telephone receiver holders are good substitutes for holding the receiver in the hand. Commercially recorded books and Talking Books (See Chapter 10, "VISION LOSS," National Library Service for the Blind and Physically Handicapped) enable individuals with visual problems to continue reading.

Individuals should wear shoes with leather soles which slide easily and avoid wearing rubber or crepe soled shoes which may cause falls when walking with shuffling steps or "freezing" due to bradykinesia.

REFERENCES

Dogali, M. et al.
1995 "Stereotactic Ventral Pallidotomy for Parkinson's Disease" NEUROLOGY 45:4(April):753-61

Duvoisin, Roger C. and Jacob Sage
1996 PARKINSON'S DISEASE: A GUIDE FOR PATIENT AND FAMILY Hagerstown, MD: Lippincott-Raven Publishers

Food and Drug Administration
2002 "FDA Approves Expanded Use of Brain Implant for Parkinson's Disease" FDA TALK PAPER January 14

Freed, Curt R. et al.
1992 "Survival of Implanted Fetal Dopamine Cells and Neurologic Improvement 12 to 46 Months after Transplantation for Parkinson's Disease" NEW ENGLAND JOURNAL OF MEDICINE 327:22(November 26):1549-55

Koller, William C.
1992 "When Does Parkinson's Disease Begin?" NEUROLOGY (April, Suppl 4):27-31

Lieberman, Abraham N. et al.
1993 PARKINSON'S DISEASE: THE COMPLETE GUIDE FOR PATIENTS AND CAREGIVERS New York, NY: Simon and Schuster

Movement Disorder Society
2002 "Commentary: When Should COMT Inhibitors be Added: Early or Late?" MOVING ALONG 4:1:4-6

National Institute of Neurological Disorders and Stroke
2001 PARKINSON'S DISEASE: HOPE THROUGH RESEARCH Bethesda, MD: National Institute of Neurological Disorders and Stroke www.ninds.nih.gov/health_and_medical/disorders/parkinsons_disease.htm

National Parkinson Foundation, Inc.
1998 "Mitochondrial Function and Coenzyme Q10 in PD" PARKINSON REPORT Miami, FL: National Parkinson Foundation

Phillips, Pat
1999 "Keeping Depression at Bay Helps Patients with Parkinson's Disease" JAMA 282:12(September 22/29):1118-1119

Spencer, Dennis D. et al.

1992 "Unilateral Transplantation of Human Fetal Mesencephalic Tissue into the Caudate Nucleus of Patients with Parkinson's Disease" NEW ENGLAND JOURNAL OF MEDICINE 327:22(November 26):1541-1548

Stern, Matthew B. and Carol A. Mackenzie

1991 "The Challenge of Young Onset PD" PARKINSON REPORT 12:4:8-9 Miami, FL: National Parkinson Foundation

ORGANIZATIONS

AMERICAN ASSOCIATION OF NEUROLOGICAL SURGEONS
5550 Meadowbrook Drive
Rolling Meadows, IL 60088
(888) 566-2267   (847) 378-0500
FAX (847) 378-0600   www.neurosurgery.com

This professional membership organization's web site offers links to "Find a Neurosurgeon" and "Health Resources" (click on Parkinson's disease).

AMERICAN PARKINSON DISEASE ASSOCIATION (APDA)
1250 Hylan Boulevard, Suite 4B
Staten Island, NY 10305
(800) 223-2732   (718) 981-8001
FAX (718) 981-4399   www.apdaparkinson.com

Sponsors information and referral centers, support groups, and research. Quarterly newsletter, "APDA Newsletter," FREE. Also available on the web site.

BRAIN RESOURCES AND INFORMATION NETWORK (BRAIN)
National Institute of Neurological Disorders and Stroke (NINDS)
PO Box 5801
Bethesda, MD 20824
(800) 352-9424   FAX (301) 402-2186
www.ninds.nih.gov

This clearinghouse distributes fact sheets and brochures about neurological disorders such as Parkinson's disease to individuals and their families. FREE

MEDLINEPLUS: PARKINSON'S DISEASE
www.nlm.nih.gov/medlineplus/parkinsonsdisease.html

This web site provides links to sites for general information about Parkinson's disease, symptoms and diagnosis, specific conditions/aspects, treatment, organizations, and research. Includes two interactive tutorials, "Parkinson's Disease" and "Pallidotomy." Some information is available in Spanish. Provides links to MEDLINE research articles and related MEDLINEplus pages.

MICHAEL J. FOX FOUNDATION FOR PARKINSON'S RESEARCH
Grand Central Station
PO Box 4777
New York, NY 10163
(800) 708-7644   www.michaeljfox.org

The foundation raises funds and awards grants for new and innovative research.

NATIONAL INSTITUTE OF NEUROLOGICAL DISORDERS AND STROKE (NINDS)
31 Center Drive, MSC 2540
Building 31, Room 8A06
Bethesda, MD 20892
(800) 352-9424   (301) 496-5751
FAX (301) 402-2186   www.ninds.nih.gov

A federal agency which conducts basic and clinical research on the causes and treatment of disorders of the brain and nervous system, including Parkinson's disease. Accepts some patients for experimental drug trials.

NATIONAL PARKINSON FOUNDATION
1501 NW 9th Avenue, Bob Hope Road
Miami, FL 33136
(800) 327-4545   (305) 547-6666
FAX (305) 243-4403   www.parkinson.org

California office:
1500 San Pablo Street
Los Angeles, CA 90033
In CA, (800) 522-8855   (323) 442-8434

New York office:
10 Union Square East, Suite 5L
New York, NY 10003
(212) 844-6050   FAX (212) 844-6056

Provides research support, diagnostic and clinical services, therapy, support groups, and outreach programs to individuals and professionals. Quarterly newsletter, "The Parkinson Report," FREE. Also available on the web site. Membership, $25.00. Clinical trials currently underway are listed on the web site. Publications are also available on the web site.

PARKINSON'S DISEASE FOUNDATION (PDF)
710 West 168th Street
New York, NY 10032
(800) 457-6676   (212) 923-4700
FAX (212) 923-4778   www.pdf.org

Provides education, counseling, advocacy, research support, and referrals for individuals, families, and professionals. Quarterly newsletter, "The PDF News," FREE.

WE MOVE (Worldwide Education and Awareness for Movement)
204 West 84th Street
New York, NY 10024
(800) 437-6682)   (212) 875-8312
www.wemove.org

This organization provides information about the management and treatment of neurological movement disorders, including

Parkinson's disease. The web site offers information for patients, professionals, and the public such as "Ask the Expert," chat rooms, and links to support and advocacy organizations.

PUBLICATIONS

BE ACTIVE! A SUGGESTED EXERCISE PROGRAM FOR PEOPLE WITH PARKINSON'S DISEASE
American Parkinson Disease Association
1250 Hylan Boulevard, Suite 4B
Staten Island, NY 10305
(800) 223-2732   (718) 981-8001
FAX (718) 981-4399   www.apdaparkinson.com

This booklet suggests a series of simple exercises aimed at making everyday tasks easier. FREE. Also available on the web site.

CARING FOR THE PARKINSON PATIENT
by J. Thomas Hutton and Raye Lynne Dippel (eds.)
Prometheus Books
59 John Glenn Drive
Amherst, NY 14228
(800) 421-0351   FAX (716) 691-0137
www.prometheusbooks.com

This book provides practical information for patients, families, and caregivers. $22.00. Also available on 4-track audiocassette on loan from the National Library Service for the Blind and Physically Handicapped regional libraries, RC 32558. FREE

THE EXERCISE PROGRAM
by E. Richard Blonsky
710 West 168th Street
New York, NY 10032
(800) 457-6676   (212) 923-4700
FAX (212) 923-4778   www.pdf.org

This program consists of three sets of exercises, presented in a standing looseleaf binder with illustrations and two audio cassettes that provide verbal cues with music for timing. $15.00

A LIFE SHAKEN: MY ENCOUNTER WITH PARKINSON'S DISEASE
by Joel Havemann
Johns Hopkins University Press
2715 North Charles Street
Baltimore, MD 21218
(800) 537-5487   (410) 516-6900
FAX (410) 516-6998   www.press.jhu.edu/press

This book, written by a journalist who was diagnosed with the condition at age 45, describes its physical and emotional effects as well as current treatments. $24.95

LIVING WELL WITH PARKINSON'S
by Glenna Wotton Atwood
John Wiley & Sons, Inc.
Consumer Center
10475 Crosspoint Boulevard
Indianapolis, IN 46256
(877) 762-2974   FAX (800) 597-3299
www.wiley.com

Written by a woman who has Parkinson's disease, this book includes medical information, practical suggestions for everyday living, and information on nutrition, exercises, and health professionals. $16.95

LIVING WITH PARKINSON'S DISEASE
by Kathleen E. Biziere and Matthias C. Kurth
Demos Medical Publishing
386 Park Avenue South, Suite 201
New York, NY 10016
(800) 532-8663   (212) 683-0072
www.demosmedpub.com

This book focuses on the medical management of the condition, functional implications, community resources, and legal and financial problems. $24.95. Orders made on the Demos web site receive a 15% discount.

THE MIDSTAGE PATIENT EXPERIENCE OR WAITING FOR THE MAGIC MUSHROOM
by Siobhan Buckley and Margaret M. Hoehn
Parkinson's Disease Foundation
710 West 168th Street
New York, NY 10032
(800) 457-6676   (212) 923-4700
FAX (212) 923-4778   www.pdf.org

This booklet discusses progression of Parkinson's disease and accompanying lifestyle alterations. Includes chapters on depression, sexuality, and interpersonal relationships. FREE

NEUROLOGICAL DISORDERS
Brain Resources and Information Network (BRAIN)
National Institute of Neurological Disorders and Stroke (NINDS)
PO Box 5801
Bethesda, MD 20824
(800) 352-9424   (301) 496-5751
www.ninds.nih.gov

This directory lists voluntary health agencies and other patient resources. FREE

ONE STEP AT A TIME
Parkinson's Disease Foundation (PDF)
710 West 168th Street
New York, NY 10032
(800) 457-6676   (212) 923-4700
FAX (212) 923-4778   www.pdf.org

This booklet recommends simple exercises to help individuals continue with daily living activities. FREE

PARKINSON'S DISEASE: A COMPLETE GUIDE FOR PATIENTS AND FAMILIES
by William J. Weiner, Lisa M. Shulman, and Anthony E. Lang
Johns Hopkins University Press
2715 North Charles Street
Baltimore, MD 21218
(800) 537-5487   (410) 516-6900
FAX (410) 516-6998   www.press.jhu.edu/press

This book discusses the signs and symptoms of the disease, diagnosis, medical and surgical treatments, and research. Includes questions and answers section and resource list. $15.95. Also available in LARGE PRINT, $19.95.

PARKINSON'S DISEASE: A GUIDE FOR PATIENT AND FAMILY
by Roger C. Duvoisin and Jacob Sage
Lippincott Williams and Wilkins
16522 Hunters Green Parkway
Hagerstown, MD 21740
(800) 638-3030   FAX (301) 223-2398
www.lww.com

This book describes Parkinson's disease, its symptoms, treatment, and methods of coping. A glossary and guide to drug treatments are included. $29.95

PARKINSON'S DISEASE: A SELF-HELP GUIDE
by Marjan Jahanshahi and David Marsden
Demos Medical Publishing
386 Park Avenue South, Suite 201
New York, NY 10016
(800) 532-8663   (212) 683-0072
www.demosmedpub.com

This book describes the diagnosis and prognosis of the condition; medical and surgical treatment; and living and coping with it. It also discusses chronic disease from the perspective of both patient and family and presents strategies for self-help and emotional well-being. $24.95. Orders made on the Demos web site receive a 15% discount.

PARKINSON'S DISEASE: FIGHTING LIKE A TIGER, THINKING LIKE A FOX
by Abraham N. Lieberman
Jones & Bartlett
40 Tall Pine Drive
Sudbury, MA 01776
(978) 443-5000   www.jbpub.com

Written by a neurologist, this book uses individual personal stories to discuss the diagnosis and treatment of the condition and strategies for living with it. Includes chapters on depression, anxiety, and dementia. $18.95

PARKINSON'S DISEASE: FITNESS COUNTS
by Rose Wichmann and Maria Waide-Douglas
National Parkinson Foundation
1501 NW 9th Avenue, Bob Hope Road
Miami, FL 33136
(800) 327-4545   (305) 547-6666
FAX (305) 243-4403   www.parkinson.org

This manual describes the role of exercise in treating individuals with Parkinson's disease. Includes illustrated exercises and recommendations for environmental modifications for safety at home and at work. FREE. Also available on the web site.

PARKINSON'S DISEASE: NUTRITION MATTERS
by Kathrynne Holden
National Parkinson Foundation
1501 NW 9th Avenue, Bob Hope Road
Miami, FL 33136
(800) 327-4545   (305) 547-6666
FAX (305) 243-4403   www.parkinson.org

This manual discusses the importance of good nutrition for individuals with Parkinson's disease. Provides sample menus and a shopping list. FREE. Also available on the web site.

PARKINSON'S DISEASE: QUESTIONS AND ANSWERS
by Robert A. Hauser and Theresa A. Zesiewicz
Merit Publishing International
8260 NW 49th Manor
Coral Springs, FL 33067
(954) 755-4280   FAX (954) 755-4287
www.meritpublishing.com

This book provides information about the diagnosis and treatment of the disease. Includes information on complications of long term therapy and management of secondary symptoms such as dysphasia, incontinence, and constipation. $29.95

PARKINSON'S DISEASE: SPEAKING OUT
by Stefanie Countryman and Janet Schwantz
National Parkinson Foundation
1501 NW 9th Avenue, Bob Hope Road
Miami, FL 33136
(800) 327-4545   (305) 547-6666
FAX (305) 243-4403   www.parkinson.org

This manual describes the effects of Parkinson's disease on speech, voice, and swallowing function and recommends strategies and exercises for maintaining communication skills. FREE. Also available on the web site.

PATIENT PERSPECTIVES ON PARKINSON'S
by Sid and Donna Dorros
National Parkinson Foundation
1501 NW 9th Avenue, Bob Hope Road
Miami, FL 33136
(800) 327-4545   (305) 547-6666
FAX (305) 243-4403   www.parkinson.org

Written by a man with Parkinson's disease and his wife, this book of essays covers medical issues and issues affecting everyday living. FREE. Also available on the web site.

PREVENTING FALLS: A DEFENSIVE APPROACH
by J. Thomas Hutton
Prometheus Books
59 John Glenn Drive
Amherst, NY 14228
(800) 421-0351   FAX (716) 691-0137
www.prometheusbooks.com

This book describes the Defensive Falls School, a program designed to help individuals with Parkinson's disease and others who are at risk for falls. Discusses topics such as vision, balance, gait, posture, and freezing; provides home safety assessments and transfer techniques; and suggests environmental changes. $19.00. A videotape that demonstrates preventive strategies is also available. 60 minutes. $22.00

SAVING MILLY: LOVE, POLITICS, AND PARKINSON'S DISEASE
by Morton Kondracke
Perseus Books Group
Customer Service Department
5500 Central Avenue
Boulder, CO 80301
(800) 386-5656   www.perseuspublishing.com

In this biography, political commentator Kondracke describes his wife's diagnosis of Parkinson's disease and its effect on their relationship and family as well as the political realities in the struggle for research funding. $25.00

300 TIPS FOR MAKING LIFE WITH PARKINSON'S DISEASE EASIER
by Shelley Peterman Schwarz
Demos Medical Publishing
386 Park Avenue South, Suite 201
New York, NY 10016
(800) 532-8663   (212) 683-0072
www.demosmedpub.com

This book contains tips, techniques, and shortcuts that enable readers to conserve energy and time and make life easier. $18.95. Orders made on the Demos web site receive a 15% discount.

254

UNDERSTANDING PARKINSON'S DISEASE: A SELF HELP GUIDE
by David L. Cram
Addicus Books, Inc.
PO Box 45327
Omaha, Ne 68145
(800) 352-2873   (402) 330-7493
FAX (402) 330-7493   www.AddicusBooks.com

Written by a physician who has Parkinson's disease, this book describes the symptoms, stages, diagnosis, and treatment of the condition and discusses the emotional aspects and day-to-day coping. Includes a chapter on caring for caregivers, glossary, bibliography, and resource list. $14.95

Chapter 9

STROKE

Stroke is a vascular disease which affects the arteries of the central nervous system. The technical term for a stroke is cerebrovascular accident (CVA). Strokes occur when a blood vessel either bursts or becomes clogged with a blood clot. A stroke stops the flow of blood that brings oxygen and nutrients to the brain. When brain cells die, they are not replaceable. The effects of stroke may be slight or severe, temporary or permanent. The behavior of stroke patients will differ, depending upon the portion of the brain that has been injured, the type of injury, the severity of the injury, and how recently the stroke occurred (Fowler and Fordyce: 1989).

In the United States, stroke is the third leading cause of death, after heart disease and cancer; however, the death rate from stroke declined by 17.3% from 1985 to 1995.

The southeastern section of the United States has become known as the stroke belt, as death from stroke is higher than the national average for both sexes and all races. People living in this region are more likely to be overweight and have high blood pressure than those in other parts of the country. The highest rate of stroke occurs among African Americans (National Heart, Lung, and Blood Institute: 1993).

There are an estimated 600,000 new and recurrent episodes of stroke each year in the United States. The incidence of stroke is decreasing, in part due to education about improving blood pressure and cholesterol through modification of diet and exercise as well as warnings about the health hazards of smoking. As the older population increases and as more individuals receive immediate post-stroke medical attention, the number of stroke survivors is increasing (Duncan: 1994). There are about 4.4 million stroke survivors in the United States (Agency for Healthcare Research and Quality: 2002).

Stroke is a major cause of long term disability. In 1993, medical and rehabilitation costs of stroke along with lost productivity cost Americans 30 billion dollars (Matchar and Duncan: 1994).

The incidence of stroke in men is about 19% higher than in women (American Heart Association: 1998). Other risk factors for stroke include race, a prior stroke, diabetes mellitus, and heredity. The risk factors associated with heart disease which increase the risk of stroke include smoking, elevated blood cholesterol, and high blood pressure and are all amenable to treatment. High blood pressure, the strongest risk factor for stroke, may be treated with diet and medication. African Americans have a greater risk of stroke due to a greater incidence of high blood pressure. Physical inactivity, another risk factor, can be changed through an exercise program.

The warning signals which may indicate a stroke include sudden weakness or numbing of the face, arm, or leg on one side of the body; a loss of speech, difficulty speaking, or understanding speech; dimness or loss of vision, particularly in one eye only; unexplained dizziness, unsteadiness, or sudden falls; or transient ischemic attacks (described below). Stroke requires immediate care. The diagnosis of stroke is confirmed through a neurological exam, computed tomography (CT scan), arteriography, digitized intravenous arteriography (DIVA), or ultrasonography.

About one-fifth to one-quarter of individuals who have had a stroke experience second or third strokes. These sometimes can be prevented with surgery and drugs. Surgery may remove built-up plaque in arteries or bypass ruptured blood vessels in the brain. Several large studies have shown that individuals with symptomatic carotid artery blockage (stenosis) of 70% or more benefit from carotid endarterectomy (American Heart Association: 1998). The reduction in the risk of stroke in individuals with 50 to 69% blockage was only moderate (Barnett et al.: 1998). Surgery was of no benefit to individuals who had less than 50% stenosis.

Drug therapy with anticoagulants such as heparin, warfarin, or aspirin may prevent new clots from forming, or prevent existing clots from becoming larger.

The effects and complications of ischemic stroke are minimized by early treatment with tissue plasminogen activator (tPA), a drug that dissolves the clot that reduces blood flow to the brain. Antiplatelet therapy (platelets are small structures in the blood concerned with blood coagulation and the contraction of blood clots) has recently been touted as a preventative measure for those who have already experienced a stroke or a stroke precursor, such as a TIA. Both ticlopidine hydrochloride and aspirin appear to be effective in preventing thrombotic strokes in individuals who have had minor strokes or TIAs and have undergone carotid endarterectomy (Easton: 1995). Although ticlopidine hydrochloride is recommended for patients who cannot tolerate aspirin, it too has side effects. Because ticlopidine may cause neutropenia, a deficiency in the blood, complete blood counts should be taken every two weeks during the first three months of therapy. In addition, possible side effects include skin rash and diarrhea (Atkinson: 1995). Ticlopidine is most effective in the first year following stroke, when the probability of recurrence is also greatest (Biller et al.: 1994).

According to Baldwin and Vacek (1989), careful monitoring of any drug therapy is especially important in elders due to variable drug absorption rates, interactions of drugs, metabolism, and excretion. The stroke survivor who participates in the management of hypertension by using a blood pressure monitor and recording readings in a daily diary provides valuable information to the physician who can adjust medications, if necessary. Self-monitoring also gives stroke survivors a sense of control over one risk factor for secondary stroke (Ozer: 1992).

Balloon angiography and stenting, common procedures in the

treatment of coronary artery disease, are now being investigated in clinical trials as possible techniques to keep carotid arteries open and avoid restenosis (Cleveland Clinic: 1998).

TYPES OF STROKE

There are two major types of strokes: ISCHEMIC STROKES, which are caused by a blood clot that results in an insufficient flow of blood to the brain, and HEMORRHAGIC STROKES, in which a blood vessel breaks and leaks into the brain.

Within each of the two major types of strokes are two types of strokes. CEREBRAL THROMBOSIS and CEREBRAL EMBOLISM are both ischemic strokes and account for 70 to 80% of all strokes (American Heart Association: 1994). In the cerebral thrombosis, a blood clot forms in the artery which brings blood to the brain or in a blood vessel in the brain itself. Clots form in arteries which are damaged by atherosclerosis (hardening of the arteries). A cerebral thrombosis usually occurs at night or first thing in the morning, when blood pressure is low.

Individuals may be forewarned of potential cerebral thrombotic strokes by experiencing TRANSIENT ISCHEMIC ATTACKS (TIAs), which may occur days, weeks, or even months before a major stroke. In a TIA, a blood clot temporarily clogs an artery, interrupting the flow of blood to a part of the brain. Symptoms, such as a loss of mobility in a hand or foot, vertigo, vision or hearing loss, occur rapidly and usually last a short time (24 hours or less). Individuals who experience TIAs are 9.5 times more likely to have a stroke than people of the same age and sex who have not had a TIA (American Heart Association: 1994). The main distinctions between a TIA and a stroke are the TIA's short duration and lack of permanent damage.

In the cerebral embolism, the bloodstream carries a blood clot to the artery leading to the brain or into the brain itself. These clots arise from diseased areas of the heart.

CEREBRAL HEMORRHAGE and SUBARACHNOID HEMORRHAGE are the two types of hemorrhagic strokes. In a cerebral hemorrhage, a blood vessel within the brain, usually an artery, ruptures. This form of stroke is associated with high blood pressure in 70% of the cases. A study revealed that low estrogen levels in women are related to this particular type of stroke, which occurs twice as frequently in women as in men. Since estrogen improves both cholesterol levels and blood pressure, it may contribute to reducing the probability of stroke (National Institutes of Health: 1994).

Subarachnoid hemorrhages occur when a blood vessel on the surface of the brain ruptures and bleeds into the space between the brain and the skull. Subarachnoid hemorrhages may be caused by head injury or burst aneurysms (blood-filled pouches that balloon out from weak areas in blood vessels).

EFFECTS OF STROKE

Of the 4.4 million stroke survivors in the United States, 15 to 30% have permanent disabilities of varying degrees and types (Agency for Healthcare Research and Quality: 2002). The effects of stroke are more severe for individuals age 65 or over; they experience twice the disability and four times the limitations in activities of daily living as those age 45 to 64 (Evans et al.: 1994).

Paralysis or weakness on one side of the body is usually the most visible sign of stroke. When one side of the body is affected, there is an injury to the opposite side of the brain. For example, paralysis on the right side of the body, or right hemiplegia, means that there is an injury to the left side of the brain. The individual with a right hemiplegia is apt to have APHASIA, which affects the ability to express thoughts and understand what is said or written by others. In expressive aphasia, speech is slow and labored, and words connecting nouns and verbs are often missing; the individual is aware of his or her difficulties. In receptive aphasia, the person has difficulty understanding speech and in monitoring his or her own conversation; he or she is often unaware of these difficulties. Global aphasia consists of both expressive and receptive aphasia (Zezima: 1994). Individuals with aphasia often have a weakness in the right arm and leg. Vision may also be affected, and in some instances, seizures may occur. DYSARTHRIA is the term used to describe the speech problems that occur when muscles in the tongue, palate, and lips are affected. Speech may be slowed, slurred, or distorted.

Loss of spatial-perceptual skills is often the result of a stroke affecting the right side of the brain and producing left hemiplegia. The ability to judge size, distance, rate of movement, and position is affected. Individuals may have trouble steering a wheelchair through a doorway, may confuse left and right, miss buttons, or lose their place when reading.

Many individuals who have had a stroke lose some of their visual field; individuals with right hemiplegia lose right field vision in both eyes, individuals with left hemiplegia lose left visual fields in both eyes. Although many individuals learn to turn their heads to compensate, some do not. This failure to compensate is called NEGLECT. Neglect can also affect all the senses on one side of the body; individuals may not recognize their own left or right arms and legs as part of their bodies. They act as though they were selectively ignoring all that happens on the impaired side.

In many individuals, the loss of function of upper extremities may be more of a problem than loss of lower extremity function. Range of motion, or the extent to which a joint can be extended and flexed, may be maintained through the use of a sling, support pillow, armboard, or medication, but it is important to use only the adaptive equipment which is actually needed.

Changes in individuals' behavior may also be attributable to stroke. The term QUALITY CONTROL is used to describe the ability to guide and check one's own behavior, sometimes known as social judgment. Individuals may become aggressive or uncommunicative, may neglect personal hygiene, or swear inappropriately. Gentle coaching, appropriate feedback, and simple memory cues may help individuals with these memory defects.

Memory problems occur with almost any injury to the brain and can have language and spatial-perceptual components. RETENTION SPAN is a term used to describe the amount of information which can be retained, used, or acted upon. Short retention spans are characteristic after a stroke. Using short, concise phrases, and brief, simple messages may avoid confusing these individuals. After a stroke, individuals have difficulty with new learning, even though they are able to recall information from the past quite well. GENERALIZATION, or applying learning from one situation to another, may also be affected. Individuals with generalization problems are very sensitive to changes in their environment and may not be able to transfer skills learned in the rehabilitation program setting to the home. Rehabilitation services provided in the home may ameliorate this problem. For these individuals, it is important to discuss changes in routine and establish new routines as quickly as possible.

STROKE REHABILITATION

The key factor in stroke rehabilitation is that it must start as soon as possible. According to one source, rehabilitation should be instituted within 48 hours of hospital admission (Gibson and Caplan: 1984). Most spontaneous recovery occurs within the first four to six months after the stroke.

> To a large degree, successful rehabilitation depends on the extent of brain damage, the person's attitude, the rehabilitation team's skill, and the cooperation of family and friends (American Heart Association: 1994, 28).

The purpose of stroke rehabilitation is to reduce dependence; improve physical activity; and enable the stroke patient to be as independent and productive as possible within the limitations caused by the stroke. The standard goals of stroke rehabilitation include prevention of complications; compensation for physical and intellectual losses; minimizing social and economic loss; and maximizing independence. Early stroke care includes maintaining range of motion in the joints; preventing pressure sores; sensory stimulation; and getting out of bed as soon as possible. Over 70% of stroke survivors can become independent in activities of daily living if they receive appropriate rehabilitation (National Stroke Association: 1991).

In evaluating an individual who has had a stroke, the rehabilitation team takes into account the following characteristics: functional ability before the stroke; the social situation and the options for a return to the community; ability to cooperate with nurses and therapists; capacity to learn new material; age; and bowel and bladder (in)continence (Gibson and Caplan: 1984). Recent government guidelines recommend that the person undergo rehabilitation as long as there is evidence of progress (Gresham et al.: 1995).

Medicare and other insurance coverage place a limit on the length of time an individual who has had a stroke may spend in an acute hospital, unless there are complications. Since most individuals will benefit from rehabilitation services, they may be discharged to a hospital rehabilitation unit or to a rehabilitation hospital. Individuals who cannot afford stroke rehabilitation services may be eligible for special funding which enables individuals with brain injuries to receive treatment at rehabilitation facilities.

The rehabilitation team is also involved in discharge planning, evaluating what the individual and the family can do for themselves; what assistance must be supplied; and what resources are available through community agencies.

PSYCHOLOGICAL ASPECTS OF STROKE

In addition to the physical and mental impairments caused by a stroke, the loss of a job, reduced financial resources, and the loss of independence and sexual function may lead to loss of self-esteem and depression. Although post-stroke depression is very common, it is often overlooked by health care providers (Rusin: 1990). Because depression may interfere with motivation for rehabilitation and improved functioning, it is important that all individuals who have experienced a stroke be screened for depression.

Often, what appears to be depression is actually the result of the brain injury caused by the stroke (organic emotional lability) and characterized by little or no obvious relationship between emotions and what is happening around the individual.

Post-stroke depression may include anxiety, loss of energy, weight and appetite loss, and sleep disturbances. This depression is due to the brain's reaction to stroke as well as psychological reactions. Neurological features of stroke such as verbal and nonverbal communication problems, emotional control, and visual and auditory losses may affect the clinical assessment of depression. The health care professionals on the stroke rehabilitation team work together to determine the extent of post-stroke depression. A neuropsychological assessment should include tests of attention span, memory, language, perceptual abilities, and cognitive functions, such as problem solving and abstract thinking. The average post-stroke depression lasts less than a year (National Institute of Mental Health: 2002).

For some individuals, post-stroke depression is reduced as physical recovery progresses. Individual or group counseling, as part of the rehabilitation program or after discharge from the hospital, may enable others to adapt emotionally to their physical condition (Schwartz and Speed: 1989). Volunteer visitation programs enable stroke survivors and family members to talk with other stroke survivors. Self-help groups, such as stroke clubs, offer individuals the opportunity to discuss their physical and emotional needs and gain practical information from the experiences of others. Attendance at a day activity program for elders contributes to continuation and maintenance of skills developed through rehabilitation and offers opportunities for socializing. Anti-depressant drugs may also be prescribed after careful consideration of any associated medical conditions and risk of side effects. Anti-depressant medications are generally safe for people who have experienced a stroke (National Institute of Mental Health: 2002).

The family plays a crucial role in rehabilitation of a stroke patient. The individual's spouse may become depressed due to feelings of guilt and fear. Other symptoms apparent in caregivers include inability to sleep, social withdrawal, and marital problems. One study found that caregivers' stress increased over time, although the caregivers had not sought help for themselves (Mcnamara et al.: 1990). A spouse may become over-protective and worry about another stroke once the individual is discharged from the rehabilitation hospital. Conferences with the spouse and other family members may help to alleviate these concerns and also put the individual who has had a stroke at ease. Receipt of information from professionals and attendance at support groups for caregivers may help to alleviate some of the stress that is inevitable. A caring and able spouse or other caregiver, a supportive family, and an understanding of stroke and its consequences are important parts of a coordinated approach to care.

PROFESSIONAL SERVICE PROVIDERS

A rehabilitation evaluation involves the coordinated efforts of the neurologist, physiatrist, nurse, physical and occupational therapists, speech and language pathologist, audiologist, social worker, and psychologist. Guidelines published by the federal government suggest that one member of the rehabilitation team be the coordinator of services, establish a baseline evaluation, and keep track of the person's progress (Gresham et al.: 1995).

NEUROLOGISTS are physicians who specialize in diagnosing and treating disorders of the brain.

PHYSIATRISTS, physicians who specialize in rehabilitation medicine, often act as case managers or team leaders, coordinating medical and rehabilitation services, working with the patient and the family, and arranging additional health care services if necessary.

PHYSICAL THERAPISTS help the individual to strengthen muscles and to improve balance and coordination. Mechanical aids such as braces, walkers, crutches, or canes are often used.

REHABILITATION NURSES provide day-to-day care of the patient who has had a stroke; report to the rehabilitation team on the progress of the patient; withdraw help as the patient recovers the ability to perform everyday activities in order to promote independence; and offer support to the patient's family in the hospital, outpatient clinic, and during home care visits.

OCCUPATIONAL THERAPISTS help the individual to improve hand-eye coordination and to develop skills for everyday activities, such as washing, dressing, homemaking, and recreation. Many assistive devices, such as reaching tools, built-up kitchen utensils, and writing aids are suggested by the occupational therapist. Shorter hospital stays have led to the development of home treatment programs involving stroke survivors and their families; these treatment programs are often managed by occupational therapists.

SPEECH AND LANGUAGE PATHOLOGISTS aid in the recovery or maintenance of speech or language function. After an assessment, speech and language pathologists design and implement a program to treat the individual's language difficulties. Often the test results obtained by speech and language pathologists will help the medical staff in caring for the individual with aphasia. These services are offered both in the hospital and on an out-patient basis.

AUDIOLOGISTS identify and evaluate hearing impairment; determine the need for hearing rehabilitation; decide whether or not a hearing aid will be beneficial; and select and fit the appropriate aid.

SOCIAL WORKERS meet with the individual and the family to help plan the individual's rehabilitation after release from the acute care hospital and rehabilitation programs. Social workers may also help individuals and their families with the emotional effects of stroke.

PSYCHOLOGISTS assess cognitive deficits and emotional reactions to stroke and provide supportive counseling.

WHERE TO FIND SERVICES

According to the National Stroke Association (no date), there are approximately 75 free-standing rehabilitation hospitals in the United States; many of these have voluntarily sought and received accreditation from the Commission on Accreditation of Rehabilitation Facilities (CARF). Recently, many hospitals have established in-patient rehabilitation units. These rehabilitation hospitals and units provide the services needed by individuals who have had a stroke.

The discharge plan for an individual who has had a stroke should include information about the resources available in the community. Physical therapy, occupational therapy, speech and language therapy, and audiology services may be provided by public and private clinics; local hospitals; home health agencies such as visiting nurse associations; nursing homes; state, federal, and private agencies which serve elders; Veterans Administration Medical Centers; and therapists in private practice.

Local offices of organizations such as the American Heart Association and the National Easter Seal Society, as well as independent living centers and hospitals, may sponsor stroke support groups or clubs to provide emotional and practical support to individuals who have had strokes, their families, and friends. The National Stroke Association defines a stroke support group as one which usually meets in a hospital or long term care facility and is led by a rehabilitation professional. Stroke clubs are primarily social groups run by stroke survivors without professional direction.

ASSISTIVE DEVICES AND TECHNIQUES

Individuals who have had a stroke often learn new techniques to do familiar activities. Residual paralysis or weakness, perceptual problems, vision loss, and difficulty in movement or coordination often require that the individual slow down, plan ahead, and use assistive devices to accomplish daily living activities. Special equipment may be used to give support, prevent deformity, or to replace lost abilities. Some devices are readily available in medical supply stores and through mail order catalogues (See Chapter 3, "MAKING EVERYDAY LIVING SAFER AND EASIER"), while others require a prescription from a health care professional.

In the bathroom, for example, nonskid tape should be placed on the bottom of the tub, and shower and grab bars should be installed. A hand-held shower head, soap-on-a-rope, and long-handled bath brushes will assist with bathing. A shower seat or chair with nonskid suction cups on its legs may help the individual feel more comfortable and safe.

When dressing, the individual should put the weaker arm or leg into the garment first, pull the clothing into place, and then insert the stronger arm or leg. In undressing, the opposite order should be followed. Dressing aids such as button hooks, elastic shoe laces, or zipper pulls and clothing with velcro fasteners, elastic waistbands, or snaps will help the individual dress more easily. In the kitchen, jar openers, long-handled tongs, utensils with built-up handles, and other assistive devices will make it easier for the individual to resume homemaking activities.

Adaptations of the physical environment are sometimes required to meet the individual's limitations. Simple adaptations include removing scatter rugs or shag carpets; raising chair seats with double cushions; or rearranging shelves for easy reach. Other adaptations include removing architectural barriers such as thresholds; installing ramps and handrails; and widening doorways.

Individuals who have had a stroke may use mobility aids such as four-legged walkers, canes, braces, and railings that help them to regain independent mobility to the greatest extent possible. Individuals who wish to drive should be evaluated by professionals who are expert in training for drivers with physical disabilities. Some rehabilitation hospitals or centers offer these training courses.

REFERENCES

Agency for Healthcare Research and Quality
2002   "Effectiveness and Cost-Effectiveness of Echocardiography and Carotid Imaging in Management of Stroke" EVIDENCE-BASED PRACTICE PROGRAMS Rockville, MD: Agency for Healthcare Research and Quality
American Heart Association
1998   GUIDELINES FOR CAROTID ENDARTERECTOMY Dallas, TX: American Heart Association
1994   HEART AND STROKE FACTS Dallas, TX: American Heart Association
Atkinson, Richard P.
1995   "Practical Information on the Administration of Antiplatelet Therapy" REDUCING THE ODDS OF STROKE (A special report of POSTGRADUATE MEDICINE) (February):36-39

Baldwin, Thomas and James Vacek
1989 "Use of Cardiovascular Drugs in the Elderly" POSTGRAD-UATE MEDICINE 85(April):319-330

Barnett, Henry J.M. et al.
1998 "Benefit of Carotid Endarterectomy in Patients with Symptomatic Moderate or Severe Stenosis" NEW ENGLAND JOURNAL OF MEDICINE 339:20(November):425

Biller, Jose et al.
1994 CONSENSUS AND CONTROVERSY: MEDICAL AND SURGICAL OPTIONS FOR STROKE PREVENTION New York, NY: Phase Five Communications

Cleveland Clinic
1998 "New Technique to Prevent Stroke" THE CLEVELAND CLINIC HEART ADVISOR Cleveland, OH: Cleveland Clinic

Duncan, Pamela W.
1994 "Stroke Disability" PHYSICAL THERAPY 74:399-407

Easton, J. Donald
1995 "Preventing Stroke: An Overview of Medical and Surgical Options" REDUCING THE ODDS OF STROKE (A special report of POSTGRADUATE MEDICINE) (February):7-13

Evans, R.L. et al.
1994 "Stroke: A Family Dilemma" DISABILITY AND REHABILITATION 16:3:110-118

Fowler, Roy S. and W.E. Fordyce
1989 STROKE: WHY DO THEY BEHAVE THAT WAY? Dallas, TX: American Heart Association

Gibson, Charles J. and Bruce M. Caplan
1984 "Rehabilitation of the Patient with Stroke" pp. 145-159 in T. Franklin Williams (ed.) REHABILITATION IN THE AGING New York, NY: Raven Press

Gresham, G.E. et al.

1995 POST-STROKE REHABILITATION: ASSESSMENT, REFERRAL, AND PATIENT MANAGEMENT Clinical Practice Guideline, No. 16 Rockville, MD: U.S. Department of Health and Human Services, Public Health Service, Agency for Health Care Policy and Research. AHCPR Pub. No. 95-0663

Mcnamara, Susan E. et al.

1990 "Caregiver Strain: Need for Late Poststroke Intervention" REHABILITATION PSYCHOLOGY 35:2:71-78

National Heart, Lung, and Blood Institute

1993 "National High Blood Pressure Education Program: Update on the Stroke Belt Projects" HEART MEMO (Fall):7

National Institutes of Health

1994 "Hormonal Factors May be Linked to Stroke in Females" NIH NEWS & FEATURES (September):4-5

National Institute of Mental Health

2002 DEPRESSION AND STROKE Bethesda, MD

National Stroke Association

1991 "Rehabilitation After Stroke" STROKE CLINICAL UPDATE 1:6(March):21-24

No RESOURCES FOR STROKE TREATMENT AND
date REHABILITATION

Ozer, Mark N.

1992 "Prevention of Secondary Stroke" BE STROKE SMART 9:1(Winter):5 Englewood, CO: National Stroke Association

Rusin, Michael J.

1990 "Stroke Rehabilitation: A Geropsychological Perspective" ARCHIVES OF PHYSICAL MEDICINE AND REHABILITATION 71(October):914-922

Schwartz, Joseph A. and Nancy Speed

1989 "Depression and Stroke" REHABILITATION REPORT 5(March-April):1-3

Zezima, Michele and Michael
1994 "Louder than Words: Treating Aphasia and Agnosia"
        ADVANCE/REHABILITATION 3 (September)8:27-28

ORGANIZATIONS

AMERICAN SPEECH-LANGUAGE-HEARING ASSOCIATION (ASHA)
10801 Rockville Pike
Rockville, MD 20852
(800) 638-8255   FAX (301) 897-7355
www.asha.org

A professional organization of speech-language pathologists and audiologists. Toll-free HELPLINE offers answers to questions about conditions and services as well as referrals. Provides information on communication problems and a FREE list of certified audiologists and speech therapists for each state. Also available on the web site. Web site also lists self-help groups for individuals with speech and language disorders.

AMERICAN STROKE ASSOCIATION
7272 Greenville Avenue
Dallas, TX 75231
(888) 478-7653   (214) 373-6300
FAX (214) 706-1341   www.strokeassociation.org

Affiliated with the American Heart Association, this organization promotes research and education and publishes professional and public education brochures. Callers can speak to stroke survivors or receive a referral to a local support group. Publishes "Stroke Connection Magazine." FREE. Publications listed on web site; will send up to 10 publications FREE.

BRAIN RESOURCES AND INFORMATION NETWORK (BRAIN)
National Institute of Neurological Disorders and Stroke (NINDS)
PO Box 5801
Bethesda, MD 20824
(800) 352-9424   FAX (301) 402-2186
www.ninds.nih.gov

This clearinghouse distributes fact sheets and brochures about neurological disorders such as stroke to individuals and their families. FREE

COMMISSION ON ACCREDITATION OF REHABILITATION FACILITIES (CARF)
4891 East Grant Road
Tucson, AZ 85712
(520) 325-1044 (V/TTY)   FAX (520) 318-1129
www.carf.org

Conducts site evaluations and accredits organizations that provide rehabilitation, pain management, adult day services, and assisted living. Provides a FREE list of accredited organizations in a specific state.

MEDLINEPLUS: SPEECH AND COMMUNICATION DISORDERS
www.nlm.nih.gov/medlineplus/
speechcommunicationsdisorders.html
MEDLINEPLUS: STROKE
www.nlm.nih.gov/medlineplus/stroke.html

These web sites provide links to sites for general information about speech and communication disorders and stroke, including symptoms and diagnosis, specific conditions/aspects, organizations, clinical trials, and research. Some information is available in Spanish. Provide links to MEDLINE research articles and related MEDLINEplus pages.

NATIONAL APHASIA ASSOCIATION
29 John Street, Suite 1103
New York, NY 10038
(800) 922-4622   (212) 267-2812
www.aphasia.org

Promotes public awareness, publishes public education brochures, and develops community programs for people with aphasia. Maintains list of health care professionals who will make referrals to local resources. Publishes a variety of inexpensive fact sheets and "Aphasia Community Group Manual," for organizers of local aphasia support groups, $30.00. Membership, $25.00, includes quarterly newsletter.

NATIONAL EASTER SEAL SOCIETY
230 West Monroe Street, Suite 1800
Chicago, IL 60606
(800) 221-6827   (312) 726-6200
(312) 726-4258 (TTY)   FAX (312) 726-1494
www.easter-seals.org

Promotes research, education, and rehabilitation for people with physical disabilities and speech and language problems. Sponsors Easter Seal Stroke Clubs for people who have had strokes, their families, and friends.

NATIONAL HEART, LUNG, AND BLOOD INSTITUTE (NHLBI)
31 Center Drive, MSC 2480
Bethesda, MD 20892
(301) 496-5166   www.nhlbi.nih.gov.

Conducts research and national education programs and issues clinical guidelines on topics such as high blood pressure and high cholesterol. Publications list available, FREE. Many publications are available on the web site.

NATIONAL HEART, LUNG, AND BLOOD INSTITUTE INFORMATION NET
PO Box 30105
Bethesda, MD 20824-0105
(800) 575-9355   (301) 592-8573
(240) 629-3255 TTY   FAX (301) 592-8563
www.nhlbi.nih.gov/health/infoctr/index.htm

A federal information center which distributes publications about cardiovascular disease. NHLBI Information Line provides recorded messages in English and Spanish about prevention and treatment of high blood pressure; [(800) 575-9355]. FREE publications list.

NATIONAL HYPERTENSION ASSOCIATION
324 East 30th Street
New York, NY 10016
(212) 889-3557   FAX (212) 447-7032
www.nathypertension.org

Conducts research, promotes public and professional education, and provides hypertension work-site detection programs. General information packet, FREE.

NATIONAL INSTITUTE OF NEUROLOGICAL DISORDERS AND STROKE (NINDS)
31 Center Drive, MSC 2540
Building 31, Room 8A06
Bethesda, MD 20892
(800) 352-9424   (301) 496-5751
FAX (301) 402-2186   www.ninds.nih.gov

A federal agency that conducts basic and clinical research on the causes, prevention, and treatment of stroke.

**NATIONAL INSTITUTE ON DEAFNESS AND OTHER COMMUNICA-
TION DISORDERS (NIDCD)**
Building 31, Room 3C35
31 Center Drive, MSC 2320
Bethesda, MD 20892
(301) 496-7243   (301) 402-0252 (TTY)
www.nidcd.nih.gov

A federal agency that funds basic research studies on problems
of hearing, balance, voice, language, and speech.

**NATIONAL INSTITUTE ON DEAFNESS AND OTHER
COMMUNICATION DISORDERS INFORMATION CLEARINGHOUSE**
1 Communication Avenue
Washington, DC 20892
(800) 241-1044   (800) 241-1055 (TTY)
FAX (301) 907-8830   www.nidcd.nih.gov

Maintains a database of references and responds to requests for
information from the public and professionals on communication
disorders including aphasia. Publishes newsletter, "Inside NIDCD
Clearinghouse." FREE

NATIONAL STROKE ASSOCIATION
9707 East Easter Lane
Englewood, CO 80112
(800) 787-6537   (303) 649-9299
FAX (303) 649-1328   www.stroke.org

Assists individuals with stroke and educates their families,
physicians, and the general public about stroke. Membership,
$25.00. Publishes bimonthly newsletter, "Stroke Smart," $12.00.
Publications are available on the web site.

RADIOLOGICAL SOCIETY OF NORTH AMERICA (RSNA)
820 Jorie Boulevard
Oak Brook, IL 60523
(630) 571-2670   FAX (630) 571-7837
www.rsna.org

Web site contains patient information, including information about diagnostic imaging techniques.

SOCIETY FOR NEUROSCIENCE (SFN)
11 Dupont Circle, Suite 500
Washington, DC 20036
(202) 462-6088   FAX (202) 234-9770
www.sfn.org

A multidisciplinary society of professionals who study the brain and the nervous system, including stroke and aphasia. Holds an annual meeting. Publishes the "Journal of Neuroscience" twice a month. A number of publications for the public, including "Neuroscience Newsletter," "Brain Briefings," and "Brain Backgrounders" are available on the web site. FREE

STROKE CONNECTION
American Stroke Association
7272 Greenville Avenue
Dallas, TX 75231
(888) 478-7653   www.strokeassociation.org

Coordinates a network of more than 1200 stroke clubs and groups. The Stroke Group Registry provides referrals to these groups; (800) 553-6321. Sponsors "Common Threads PenFriends," which matches stroke survivors, caregivers, and family members. Bimonthly newsletter, "Stroke Connection Magazine," FREE.

PUBLICATIONS AND TAPES

AGING: YOU SHOULD LIVE SO LONG
The Kids on the Block
9385-C Gerwig Lane
Columbia, MD 21046
(800) 368-5437   (410) 290-9095
FAX (410) 290-9358   www.kotb.com

A program designed to help children and adults understand the nature of aging and disabilities. Uses puppets to act out roles in script, including a grandmother who is recovering from a stroke and her grandson. Program, which includes teacher's guide, scripts, and questions and answers, $250.00; puppets additional.

APHASIA
National Institute on Deafness and Other Communication Disorders Information Clearinghouse
1 Communication Avenue
Washington, DC 20892
(800) 241-1044   (800) 241-1055 (TTY)
FAX (301) 907-8830   www.nidcd.nih.gov

This fact sheet describes the causes of aphasia, diagnosis, and treatment. Includes resource list. FREE. Also available on the web site.

APHASIA, MY WORLD ALONE
by Helen Harlan Wulf
Wayne State University Press
4809 Woodward Avenue
Detroit, MI 48201
(800) 978-7323   (313) 577-6120
FAX (313) 577-6131   www.wsupress.wayne.edu

The author shares the experience of her stroke and aphasia, with emphasis on speech therapy, family relationships, and the effects of fatigue on recovery. $14.95

BRAIN ATTACKS
Aquarius Health Care Videos
Olde Medfield Square
266 Main Street, Suite 33B
Medfield, MA 02052
(888) 440-2963   FAx (508) 242-9854
www.aquariusproductions.com

This videotape describes the risk factors, warning signals and treatment available for stroke. Includes personal accounts of stroke survivors. 30 minutes. $195.00

CARING FOR A PERSON WITH APHASIA
American Heart Association
7272 Greenville Avenue
Dallas, TX 75231
(800) 242-8721   (214) 373-6300
FAX (214) 706-1341   www.americanheart.org

This booklet describes the communication problems associated with aphasia and provides practical tips for improving communication skills. FREE

COPING WITH APHASIA
by Jon C. Lyon
Thomson Learning
7625 Empire Drive
Florence, KY 41042
(800) 347-7707   FAX (859) 647-5023
www.thomsonlearning.com

This book deals with the causes and medical treatments of aphasia as well as the emotional aspects. $53.00

DIRECTORY: INFORMATION RESOURCES FOR HUMAN COMMUNICATION DISORDERS
National Institute on Deafness and Other Communication Disorders Information Clearinghouse
1 Communication Avenue
Washington, DC 20892
(800) 241-1044   (800) 241-1055 (TTY)
FAX (301) 907-8830   www.nidcd.nih.gov

This directory provides a listing and description of organizations throughout the country that deal with communication disorders. FREE. Also available on the web site.

LOOKIN' FOR ME
National Aphasia Association
29 John Street, Suite 1103
New York, NY 10038
(800) 922-4622   (212) 267-2812
www.aphasia.org

This videotape features interviews with three individuals with aphasia. It emphasizes how to communicate with people who have aphasia. 22 minutes. $10.00

LOWERING BLOOD PRESSURE
National Heart, Lung, and Blood Institute Information Net
PO Box 30105
Bethesda, MD 20824-0105
(800) 575-9355   (301) 592-8573
(240) 629-3255 TTY   FAX (301) 592-8563
www.nhlbi.nih.gov/health/infoctr/index.htm

This booklet provides information about how blood pressure affects health and measures to take to lower it. FREE

MANAGING STROKE: A GUIDE TO LIVING WELL AFTER STROKE
by Paul R. Rao, Mark N. Ozer, and John E. Toerge (eds.)
National Rehabilitation Hospital
102 Irving Street, NW
Washington, DC 20010
(202) 877-1776   (202) 829-5180
www.nrhrehab.org

This book provides information on the medical, financial, and psychological aspects of living with stroke. Includes guidance for choosing a rehabilitation program. $13.95

NEUROLOGICAL DISORDERS
Brain Resources and Information Network (BRAIN)
National Institute of Neurological Disorders and Stroke (NINDS)
PO Box 5801
Bethesda, MD 20824
(800) 352-9424   (301) 496-5751
www.ninds.nih.gov

This directory lists voluntary health agencies and other patient resources. FREE

ONE HAND CAN DO THE WORK OF TWO
A/V Health Services
PO Box 20271
Roanoke, VA 24018-0028
(540) 986-3275 (Voice and FAX)
www.avhealthservices.com

This videotape shows how someone who has had a cerebral hemorrhage accomplishes household activities with the use of one hand. 20 minutes. $45.00

ONE HUNDRED QUESTIONS AND ANSWERS ABOUT HYPERTENSION
by William M. Manger and Ray W. Gifford
Blackwell Science
Commerce Place, 350 Main Street
Malden, MA 02148
(781) 388-8250   FAX (802) 864-7626
www.blackwellscience.com

Written by two physicians who specialize in the treatment of hypertension, this book provides information about the causes of hypertension and current treatments in order to enable readers to play a role in their own medical decisions. $14.95

PORTRAIT OF APHASIA
by David R. Knox
Wayne State University Press
4809 Woodward Avenue
Detroit, MI 48201
(800) 978-7323   (313) 577-6120
FAX (313) 577-6131   www.wsupress.wayne.edu

In this book, the author describes his wife's recovery from a stroke. Includes many helpful suggestions for helping individuals with aphasia regain language skills. $14.95

THE ROAD AHEAD: A STROKE RECOVERY GUIDE
National Stroke Association
9707 East Easter Lane
Englewood, CO 80112
(800) 787-6537   (303) 649-9299
FAX (303) 649-1328   www.stroke.org

This handbook helps individuals who have had strokes and their families understand the many aspects of recovering from stroke. $14.50

STROKE: HOPE THROUGH RESEARCH
National Institute of Neurological Disorders and Stroke (NINDS)
31 Center Drive, MSC 2540
Building 31, Room 8A06
Bethesda, MD 20892
(800) 352-9424   (301) 496-5751
FAX (301) 402-2186   www.ninds.nih.gov

This booklet describes the different types of stroke, diagnosis, treatment, risk factors, and current research. Also includes a glossary. FREE

A STROKE MANUAL FOR FAMILIES
HDI Publishers
PO Box 131401
Houston, TX 77219
(800) 321-7037   In TX, (713) 526-6900
FAX (713) 526-7787   www.braininjurybooks.com

This book offers suggestions for families of stroke survivors. $4.50

STROKE: QUESTIONS YOU HAVE...ANSWERS YOU NEED
by Jennifer Hay
People's Medical Society
462 Walnut Street
Allentown, PA 18102
(800) 624-8773   (610) 770-1670
FAX (610) 770-0607   www.peoplesmed.org

This book uses a question and answer format to provide information on the types of stroke, risk factors, diagnosis, treatment, and rehabilitation. Includes resources for caregivers, self-help organizations, and a glossary. $10.95

THE STROKE RECOVERY BOOK: A GUIDE FOR PATIENTS AND FAMILIES
by Kip Burkman
Addicus Books, Inc.
PO Box 45327
Omaha, Ne 68145
(800) 352-2873   (402) 330-7493
FAX (402) 330-7493   www.AddicusBooks.com

Written by a rehabilitation physician, this book describes the warning signs, causes, and types of strokes and the deficits strokes cause. It discusses cognitive and sensory impairments, speech and language disruptions, hemiplegia, dysphagia, and other medical complications. It also provides information on recovery, rehabilitation, and aftercare. $14.95

STROKE SURVIVORS
by William H. Bergquist, Rod McLean and Barbara A. Kobylinski
Jossey-Bass Publishers
San Francisco, CA

This book uses the personal histories of stroke survivors to describe the stroke experience, the recovery and rehabilitation process, and the viewpoints of caregivers. Out of print

TED'S STROKE: THE CAREGIVER'S STORY
by Ellen Paullin
National Stroke Association
9707 East Easter Lane
Englewood, CO 80112
(800) 787-6537   (303) 649-9299
FAX (303) 649-1328   www.stroke.org

This book describes personal experiences and provides guidance for caregivers of stroke survivors. $16.95

WHEN THE BRAIN GOES WRONG
by Jonathan David and Roberta Cooks
Fanlight Productions
4196 Washington Street, Suite 2
Boston, MA 02131
(800) 937-4113   (617) 469-4999
FAX (617) 469-3379   www.fanlight.com

A stroke survivor's experience is included in this videotape, which deals with seven types of brain dysfunctions. 47 minutes. Purchase, $195.00; rental for one day, $50.00; rental for one week, $100.00.

Chapter 10

VISION LOSS

Visual impairment is one of the most common impairments among the population age 65 or older. A U.S. Census Bureau survey reported that nearly four million Americans in this age category (12%) had difficulty reading letters and words in ordinary newsprint even when wearing corrective lenses; 3.3% of elders could not see letters or words at all (McNeil: 2001). Those age 85 or over experience visual impairment at higher rates; nearly one-third or 32% have visual impairments. Very few elders with visual impairments used special lenses or other devices to help them with daily activities (Desai et al: 2001).

Many elders accept vision loss and other disabilities as a "normal part of aging" and therefore do not seek out services. A study of elders living in the community (Branch et al.: 1989) found that elders with vision loss represent a population of "extensive unmet needs." This study found that elders with vision loss had difficulty carrying out the tasks of everyday living required to continue living in the community, but they did not receive adequate social services, health services, or mental health services. According to Branch and his colleagues, neither the aging service network nor the blindness system has addressed the needs of elders with vision loss adequately. Other researchers have confirmed this finding. Biegel and his associates (1989) found that few aging agencies knew how many of their clients were visually impaired or blind. A study by Stuen (1991) found that staff in 83% of the responding aging agencies felt they needed more information about visual impairment.

A study found that elders residing in nursing homes experienced blindness at rates higher than their counterparts living in the community (13 times higher for African Americans and nearly 16 times higher for whites). The authors suggested that over 40% of the blindness could be prevented or treated, most notably through cataract extraction (Tielsch et al.: 1995).

Duffy and Beliveau-Tobey (1991) observed that the high prevalence of vision loss among residents of long term care facilities has been recognized by many experts, yet little has been done to train the staff at these facilities to cope with the problem. Their national survey and test of a pilot in-service curriculum suggest that training the staff of long term care facilities can help alleviate many of the residents' problems that are associated with visual impairment.

Most elders who have experienced vision loss still retain some useful vision. Low vision is the term used to describe residual vision. The World Health Organization defines moderate low vision as an acuity of 20/70 to 20/160 in the better eye with the best possible correction. Severe low vision is defined as 20/200 to 20/400 or a visual field of 20 degrees or less (U.S. Department of Health and Human Services: 1980). "Legal blindness" is the criterion used by the federal government and most state governments to determine eligibility for vocational rehabilitation, tax exemptions, and other financial benefits. Legal blindness is defined as acuity of 20/200 or less in the better eye with the best possible correction or a field of 20 degrees or less diameter in the better eye.

MAJOR TYPES AND CAUSES OF VISION LOSS

The two major types of visual impairments are central vision loss and peripheral field loss. Central vision enables people to read, recognize faces, and to do close work. The retina is the layer at the back of the eye that acts as the eye's camera. The macula is the small central part of the retina that is responsible for acute vision. When the macula is destroyed or damaged, central vision is affected. Although individuals with macular diseases have difficulty reading or may not be able to read at all, they usually have useful peripheral vision. People with central vision loss may also have difficulty recognizing faces. For this reason, a person with macular disease may sometimes appear to be looking at another person's face out of the side of his or her eyes.

Peripheral vision is not as acute as central vision; it enables individuals to be mobile and to see the broad scope of the scene they are facing. When peripheral vision is diminished, it results in what is often referred to as tunnel vision. This impairment affects mobility, although the central vision may still be intact. Some progressive diseases, such as glaucoma, begin with loss of peripheral vision but may progress to total loss of vision, including central vision.

The three leading causes of vision loss, macular degeneration, glaucoma, and cataract, are all associated with aging. Other conditions which may lead to vision loss are stroke, diabetes, retinal detachment, trauma, and tumors.

MACULAR DEGENERATION is the term applied to a variety of diseases that cause the macula to deteriorate. The most common form of macular degeneration is age-related macular degeneration. As its name implies, this form of the disease occurs most frequently among the population age 50 or older. Age-related macular degeneration is the leading cause of vision loss among Americans age 65 or older. The disease causes loss of central vision, but some useful central vision usually remains. Symptoms of macular degeneration include distortion of straight lines or a loss of clarity in the central field of vision. For some forms of macular degeneration, laser treatment temporarily halts the progressive vision loss.

Currently there is no treatment for the drusenoid or dry form of AMD. The neovascular or wet form involves the development of abnormal blood vessels and usually causes more severe impairment than the dry form. In April, 2000, the Food and Drug Administration (FDA) approved the use of photodynamic therapy with a light-activating drug called verteporfin (Visudyne) in individuals with the wet form of AMD. However, this treatment is not able to restore vision that has already been lost. In 2001, the National Eye Institute reported the results of the Age-Related Eye

Disease Study (AREDS). In this major clinical trial, the risk of developing the more serious wet form of AMD in those who have dry AMD was reduced in participants who took antioxidants and zinc supplements (Age-Related Eye Disease Study: 2001). AMD is not cured nor is vision restored by taking the supplements.

Optical and nonoptical aids (described below) enable many elders with macular degeneration to use their remaining vision to continue reading, working, and living independently.

GLAUCOMA is a group of eye diseases in which increased intraocular pressure, caused by improper drainage of the fluid in the eye, results in damage to the optic nerve. Glaucoma is often not diagnosed until the late stages of the disease, because symptoms are not present in the early stages. When symptoms do appear, they are in the form of peripheral field defects and blurred vision. Routine ophthalmic examinations are recommended in order to detect asymptomatic diseases such as glaucoma. In addition to measuring intraocular pressure, the ophthalmologist should examine the optic nerve through dilated pupils. Progression of glaucoma can be prevented, but sight that has been lost as a result of glaucoma cannot be restored. The most common form of treatment is medication used to decrease the intraocular pressure. Medication is sometimes administered orally and sometimes applied topically as drops for the eyes. In some cases, laser treatment or microsurgery is necessary to decrease intraocular pressure.

A CATARACT is an opacity or clouding of the lens inside the eye which results in decreased visual acuity. A cataract may develop in one eye only or in both eyes at different rates. Symptoms of cataracts include blurred vision, reduced contrast sensitivity, reduced color perception, and difficulty with reading and night driving. Cataracts may be removed by surgery, which has a high success rate. When the cataract is removed, the function of the lens is usually replaced by an intraocular lens (IOL), which is placed in the eye surgically. In some individuals, the lens capsule becomes cloudy a year or more after cataract surgery (posterior capsular opacification). This condition can be treated by laser surgery, usually on an out-patient basis. Cataracts may be present with other eye diseases that cause reduced vision; thus removing a cataract does not always restore vision to normal.

PSYCHOLOGICAL ASPECTS OF VISION LOSS

A study of elders who were visually impaired or blind concluded that visual impairment that occurs later in life has enormous impact on all aspects of the individual's life. Vision loss increases elders' awareness of the decline of their physical powers and makes them intimately familiar with the incapacities of old age (Ainlay: 1989). Vision loss often occurs along with other physical disabilities:

> It is difficult for a person to mobilize strengths and compensate for the loss of vision by sharpening the use of other senses when those other senses are also deteriorating and strengths are diminishing (Associated Services for the Blind: 1988, 2).

The individual's personal and social independence is affected, influencing attitudes and emotional status, as well as the ability to adapt to loss. In addition, vision loss is responsible for many of the falls experienced by elders; the misuse of medication when labels cannot be read; and driving accidents (Wright: 1986). The loss of independence that often accompanies vision loss results in lowered self-esteem and depression. The ability to accept rehabilitation services is often delayed by the individual's need to grieve for his or her lost vision. Counseling from professional service providers and peers may help the individual to realize that others have gone through what he or she is now experiencing. Once the individual has achieved emotional acceptance of vision loss, training from rehabilitation agencies plus the use of assistive devices can enable the individual to regain his or her independence and self-esteem.

PROFESSIONAL SERVICE PROVIDERS

OPHTHALMOLOGISTS are physicians who specialize in diseases of the eye and systemic diseases that affect the eye's functioning. Ophthalmologists should refer patients for rehabilitation services when medical or surgical treatment is not effective.

OPTOMETRISTS (O.D.) are trained to conduct refractions and prescribe corrective lenses. In some states, optometrists are also licensed to administer drugs.

OPTICIANS are trained to make and dispense corrective lenses.

LOW VISION SPECIALISTS may be ophthalmologists, optometrists, opticians, or other professionals who are trained to help individuals with vision loss make use of their remaining vision to the greatest extent possible through the use of optical and nonoptical aids.

REHABILITATION COUNSELORS serve as case coordinators for elders who are visually impaired and require rehabilitation services. Rehabilitation counselors establish a one-to-one relationship through the initial interview and succeeding contacts and help the individual to establish a work plan that is appropriate, realistic, and agreed upon by the counselor and the individual (Individual Written Rehabilitation Program or IWRP). Rehabilitation guidelines have been revised to include the role of "homemaker" as a justifiable rehabilitation goal.

REHABILITATION TEACHERS provide individualized instruction in activities of daily living. This instruction may include practical adaptations such as big button telephones; markers for stoves, thermostats, and medications; and suggestions to increase home safety. Rehabilitation teachers also provide information about community resources and services.

ORIENTATION AND MOBILITY (O & M) instructors orient the individual to his or her home, the immediate areas outside the home, and commonly traveled routes. They also teach safe travel skills using the long white cane.

OCCUPATIONAL THERAPISTS are trained to assess the home, school, and work environment and to suggest environmental adaptations and assistive devices. They teach individuals with vision loss and other disabilities how to become independent in their everyday activities.

Other health professionals who may be involved in the care of individuals with vision loss are geriatricians, diabetologists, and mental health professionals such as psychologists, psychiatrists, social workers, and other counselors.

WHERE TO FIND SERVICES

Services for people with vision loss are often offered in ophthalmologists' or optometrists' offices, hospitals, and private or public rehabilitation agencies. These services include the prescription of optical and nonoptical aids which enable individuals to make maximum use of their remaining vision.

Low vision services, sometimes called low vision clinics, are operated by ophthalmologists, optometrists, or other professionals who have been specially trained in low vision. Professionals in low vision services assess their clients' visual functioning and how it affects their daily activities. Many low vision services require a referral from an ophthalmologist or optometrist along with results of a recent ophthalmological exam. Before making an appointment at a low vision service, it is wise to ask about the types of services provided. Some low vision services allow clients to borrow aids for a specified period of time prior to purchase.

Every state has an agency that provides services to individuals who are visually impaired or blind. Many telephone directories list these agencies under "Community Services Numbers" or "Government Listings." Sometimes these agencies are called "Commissions for the Blind;" they are sometimes part of the state vocational rehabilitation agency. To learn the address of a local office of the state agency, individuals should contact the information operator for the state government. Both public and private agencies offer rehabilitation services to help people continue with daily activities, such as school, work, and home-making. Some organizations offer independent living programs to elders, including low vision services, advocacy or self/advocacy training, peer counseling, and housing assistance. Most public agencies require that clients be legally blind in order to receive services. If elders do not know if they are legally blind, they should ask an ophthalmologist or optometrist. Some agencies which have the word "blind" in their names serve individuals with varying degrees of visual impairment, including low vision.

Many state agencies provide special services to elders with vision loss under the federally funded program, Independent Living Services for Older Individuals Who Are Blind, authorized by Title VII, Part C of the Rehabilitation Act as amended. Individuals must be 55 years or older in order to receive services under this program. States may provide a variety of services under this law, including visual screenings, surgical or therapeutic treatment to correct eye conditions, eyeglasses and other vision aids, aids that enable elders to be independent, mobility training, reader services, and transportation.

Obtaining appropriate rehabilitation services can prevent unnecessary placement in nursing homes and other long term care facilities. Elders living with family members may be fearful of losing their independence if their spouse or another family member becomes overly protective and tries to do everything for them. In such instances, it is often useful to seek out family counseling or to attend a self-help group that includes family members.

ADAPTATIONS FOR ELDERS WITH VISION LOSS

The following adaptations are appropriate for elders' homes, senior centers, service providers' offices, or any setting that elders frequent.

- **ENLARGE IMAGES AND OBJECTS** Increasing the size of an object projects it on to a larger part of the retina. LARGE PRINT labels for telephone dials or push-buttons are two simple examples. Hand-held and stand magnifiers are useful for reading mail, menus, price tags, telephone numbers, newspapers, and books. Closed circuit television systems (CCTVs) or video magnifiers, which enlarge print on a screen, and LARGE PRINT materials also make reading easier.

- **MOVE CLOSER** to the object by moving the body or by bringing the object closer (as when holding a book closer).

- **INCREASE THE AMOUNT OF LIGHT** Two to three times more light than usual may be necessary. Fluorescent lighting diffuses evenly and is inexpensive, but it produces less contrast, may flicker, and is harsh. Diffusing filters may solve these problems. The incandescent light of a standard bulb offers more contrast and can be directed, but it produces shadows and glare. Halogen bulbs emit a whiter light than incandescent bulbs, making reading easier; last longer; and produce more light per watt. Diffusers and additional lighting spread the light around and reduce shadows. A combination of lights is often the best choice. Sunlight is natural and bright but not easily controlled. Magnifiers with light bulbs in their handles both enlarge and illuminate print.

- **CONTROL GLARE** Glare is best controlled by dimmer switches. Night lights may help with accommodation problems, avoiding the need to turn on a bright light when rising in a dark room or walking down a dark hall.

- **INCREASE CONTRAST** The use of light/dark color combinations is important because color perception is often reduced in elders with visual impairments. It is a good idea to paint or carpet stairs in a color that contrasts with the floor above and below; to use white or light colored dishes on colored tablecloths; and to pour liquids against contrasting backgrounds. Other practical adaptations are painting stripes or placing tape in contrasting colors on the edges of steps; and marking stove and thermostat dials.

The following guidelines are useful for family members and professionals:

· Be sure that the individual knows that you are talking to him or her. Use a normal speaking voice unless you know that the individual has a hearing loss. Always look the individual in the eye when speaking.

· Use sighted guide technique: the person with vision loss holds the arm of the sighted person and follows a step behind. (An orientation and mobility instructor or a rehabilitation teacher can provide instruction in this simple technique.)

· State when you are entering or leaving the room.

· If in doubt about whether individuals need help, simply ask if they need assistance.

ASSISTIVE DEVICES

There are many useful assistive devices, ranging from the simple to complex, which help elders with vision loss to live independently. One of the simplest aids is the BOLD pen, available in stationery stores. Other simple writing aids include bold line paper and signature guides.

LARGE PRINT reading materials are very popular with elders. In addition to popular fiction works, reference books, cookbooks, bibles, and other religious materials are available in LARGE PRINT and recorded formats. Most public libraries have LARGE PRINT collections.

Telephones may be adapted with LARGE PRINT dials or push-button labels. Big button phones are available in many stores. Self-threading needles and LARGE PRINT instruction books allow elders with vision loss to continue with sewing and other hand-crafts. LARGE PRINT letters on self-adhesive tape, raised dots, and special glues may be used to label items such as canned goods, medications, and appliances. Recreational items such as playing cards, bingo cards, crossword puzzle books, and board games such as Monopoly are available in LARGE PRINT versions. LARGE PRINT or tactile watches and talking watches, clocks, thermometers, and blood glucose monitors are additional devices that help elders manage their everyday activities.

Banking is easier with LARGE PRINT checks, deposit slips, and check registers, as well as a check writing guide, which fits over a standard check and provides window guides for filling out the check. Some banks offer special services to customers with vision loss.

Many people with vision loss use "high tech" electronic aids which have been specially adapted to enhance their remaining vision. These aids include closed circuit television systems (CCTVs) and computers with LARGE PRINT, speech, or braille output. Advances in technology have resulted in the prolifer-ation of a wide variety of such aids. These aids enable people to work, keep track of their financial affairs, maintain correspon-dence, and carry out other activities that require reading and writing (See Chapter 6, High Tech Aids, in "Living with Low Vision: A Resource Guide for People with Sight Loss," listed below under "PUBLICATIONS AND TAPES" for manufacturers of these aids.).

Many public libraries and universities have established computer access centers where individuals may see the equip-ment and have "hands-on" experience before making the invest-ment in their own equipment. Some libraries will lend portable equipment to patrons.

Television is more accessible to elders with vision loss through Descriptive Video Service (DVS), which uses an additional channel to narrate a description of the actions and settings that take place in the program. It is accessible through a stereo television or a stereo VCR that includes the Second Audio Program (SAP) feature, or an SAP receiver, which is a special stereo attachment for a television. The local public broadcasting station can provide information about its DVS programming. In some areas, the DVS narration is broadcast over the local radio reading service. Popular movies with DVS narration are available for purchase, rental, or loan in video stores and public libraries. Section 713 of the Telecommunications Act of 1996 (P.L. 104-104) requires that video services be accessible to individuals with visual impairments via descriptive video services. Effective April 1, 2002, rules implemented by the Federal Communications Commission (FCC) require that television stations provide a minimum number of video described programs per quarter (www.fcc.gov). The web site www.adinternational.org provides a list of such programs on a weekly basis.

An increasing number of theatres offer first-run movies with video description accessible to patrons through headsets. In some areas, performing arts productions are also described.

Elders who can no longer read the newspaper may enjoy radio reading service broadcasts. Radio reading services are accessible through special closed channel radio receivers, stereo televisions and VCRs, and on some cable television systems. These services read local newspapers, bestsellers, and special consumer programs. The name and address of a local radio reading service is available from the state agency that provides services to individuals who are visually impaired or blind. The International Association of Audio Information Services (IAAIS), also has this information, c/o WVTF Public Radio, 4235 Electric Road, Suite 105, Roanoke, VA 24014 (800) 280-5325. www.iaais.org Some state agencies provide receivers to eligible clients; some radio reading services will provide FREE receivers.

REFERENCES

Age-Related Eye Disease Study Group
2001   "A Randomized, Placebo-controlled, Clinical Trial of High-Dose Supplementation with Vitamins C and E, Beta Carotene, and Zinc for Age-Related Macular Degeneration and Vision Loss: AREDS Report No. 8" ARCHIVES OF OPHTHALMOLOGY 119:10(October):1533-1534

Ainlay, Stephen C.
1989   DAY BROUGHT BACK MY NIGHT: AGING AND NEW VISION LOSS London and New York, NY: Routledge

Associated Services for the Blind
1988   VOLUNTEERS FOR THE VISUALLY IMPAIRED ELDERLY: A COORDINATED APPROACH TO SERVICE DELIVERY Associated Services for the Blind, 919 Walnut Street, Philadelphia, PA 19107

Biegel, David E. et al.
1989   "Unmet Needs and Barriers to Service Delivery for the Blind and Visually Impaired Elderly"   THE GERONTOLOGIST 29:1:86-91

Branch, Lawrence G., Amy Horowitz, and Cheryl Carr
1989   "The Implications for Everyday Life of Incident Self-Reported Visual Decline Among People Over Age 65 Living in the Community" THE GERONTOLOGIST 29(March):359-365

Desai, M. et al.
2001   "Trends in Vision and Hearing among Older Americans" TRENDS IN AGING No. 2 Hyattsville, MD: National Center for Health Statistics

Duffy, Maureen and Monica Beliveau-Tobey
1991   "Providing Services to Visually Impaired Elders in Long Term Care Facilities: A Multidisciplinary Approach" pp. 93-107 in Susan L. Greenblatt (ed.) MEETING THE NEEDS OF PEOPLE WITH VISION LOSS: A MULTIDISCIPLINARY PERSPECTIVE Lexington, MA: Resources for Rehabilitation

McNeil, Jack
2001   AMERICANS WITH DISABILITIES 1997: CURRENT POPULA-
        TION REPORTS P70-73 Washington, DC: U.S. Census
        Bureau
Stuen, Cynthia
1991   "Awareness of Resources for Visually Impaired Older
        Adults Among the Aging Network" JOURNAL OF GERON-
        TOLOGICAL SOCIAL WORK 17(3/4):165-179
Tielsch, James M. et al.
1995   "The Prevalence of Blindness and Visual Impairment
        Among Nursing Home Residents in Baltimore" NEW
        ENGLAND JOURNAL OF MEDICINE 332:18(May 4):1205-
        1209
U.S. Department of Health and Human Services
1980   INTERNATIONAL CLASSIFICATION OF DISEASES 9th
        Revision, Clinical Modification Volume 1 Public Health Ser-
        vice, Health Care Financing Administration
Wright, Irving S.
1986   "Keeping an Eye on the Rest of the Body" OPHTHAL-
        MOLOGY 94(September):1196-1198

ORGANIZATIONS

AD INTERNATIONAL
www.adinternational.org

This organization supports and advocates for Audio Description in movies, performing arts, videos, and television. Weekly schedule of TV programs with audio description is available on the web site.

AMD ALLIANCE INTERNATIONAL
1314 Bedford Avenue, Suite 210
Baltimore, MD 21208
(877) 263-7171   www.amdalliance.org

Offers brochure, toll-free hotline for consumers, and web site.

AMERICAN ACADEMY OF OPHTHALMOLOGY (AAO)
PO Box 7424
San Francisco, CA 94120-7424
(415) 561-8500   www.aao.org

Professional organization of ophthalmologists. Sponsors the National Eye Care Project Helpline, (800) 222-3937, which refers eligible elders for medical eye care at no out-of-pocket expense. Individuals must be 65 or older, U.S. citizens or legal residents, and not have access to an ophthalmologist they have seen in the past. Web site provides a link to "Find an Eye MD."

AMERICAN COUNCIL OF THE BLIND (ACB)
1155 15th Street, NW, Suite 1004
Washington, DC 20005
(800) 424-8666   (202) 467-5081
FAX (202) 467-5085   www.acb.org

National membership organization that provides information and advocates on behalf of individuals who are visually impaired or blind. Makes referrals to local affiliates. The toll-free number provides the "Washington Connection," a recorded message about legislation, available daily, from 5 p.m. to 9 a.m., E.S.T., and weekends. Publishes the "Braille Forum," a monthly newsletter available in alternate formats and on the web site. Membership, $5.00.

AMERICAN FOUNDATION FOR THE BLIND (AFB)
11 Penn Plaza, Suite 300
New York, NY 10001
(800) 232-5463   (212) 502-7600
FAX (212) 502-7774   www.afb.org

An information clearinghouse on blindness and visual impairment. "AFB Press Catalog of Publications," FREE. Also available on the web site. "Services Center" is a searchable database, available on the web site, where users may find service providers by name, state, country, or service category.

BLINDED VETERANS ASSOCIATION (BVA)
477 H Street, NW
Washington, DC 20001
(800) 669-7079   (202) 371-8880
www.bva.org

The BVA's field service and outreach employment programs help veterans find rehabilitation services, training, and employment. Membership, $8.00, includes the "BVA Bulletin" in LARGE PRINT and on disk. Newsletter also available on the web site.

DESCRIPTIVE VIDEO SERVICE (DVS)
WGBH
125 Western Avenue
Boston, MA 02134
Information line, (800) 333-1203
(617) 300-3600   www.dvs.wgbh.org

This organization provides descriptive video services for television programs broadcast on the Public Broadcasting System. Many local Public Broadcasting System affiliates across the country subscribe to this service; a list of these stations is available from DVS. Publishes quarterly newsletter, "DVS Guide," available in LARGE PRINT and braille; on audio through the DVS toll-free information line, (800) 333-1203; and on the Internet at the address above; FREE. For a biweekly broadcast schedule on PBS and Turner Classic Movies cable, call (800) 333-1203. Sells DVS videotapes of popular movies; call (888) 818-1999 for FREE catalogue. Special equipment is not required to hear the narration.

FEDERAL COMMUNICATIONS COMMISSION (FCC)
445 12th Street, SW
Washington, DC 20554
(888) 225-5322   (888) 835-5322 (TTY)
(202) 418-0190   (202) 418-2555 (TTY)
www.fcc.gov

Responsible for developing regulations for telecommunication issues related to federal laws, including the ADA and the Telecommunications Act of 1996.

FOUNDATION FIGHTING BLINDNESS
11435 Cronhill Drive
Owings Mills, MD 21117
(888) 394-3937   (800) 683-5551 (TTY)
(410) 568-0150   www.blindness.org

Self-help organization and information clearinghouse for individuals with retinal disorders. Local affiliates throughout the country. Supports research, retina donor program, and national retinitis pigmentosa registry. Publishes bimonthly newsletter, "Fighting Blindness News," (three full issues and three "Update" supplements) available in alternate formats and on the web site. FREE

GLAUCOMA FOUNDATION
116 John Street, Suite 1605
New York, NY 10038
(800) 452-8266   (212) 285-0080
www.glaucoma-foundation.org

Supports research into the causes and treatment of glaucoma. Operates a direct response hot-line. Publishes "Doctor, I Have a Question: A Guide for Patients and Their Families" and "Eye to Eye," a quarterly newsletter; both in LARGE PRINT. Single copies, FREE. Also available on the web site.

GLAUCOMA RESEARCH FOUNDATION
200 Pine Street, Suite 200
San Francisco, CA 94104
(800) 826-6693   (415) 986-3162
FAX (415) 986-3763   www.glaucoma.org

Offers public education programs and telephone support network. Quarterly newsletter, "Gleams," FREE; available in standard print and audiocassette (for legally blind individuals). Also available on the web site. Operates an eye donor network, which enables researchers to study the eyes donated by individuals with glaucoma and their families.

HELEN KELLER NATIONAL CENTER FOR DEAF-BLIND YOUTHS AND ADULTS (HKNC)
111 Middle Neck Road
Sands Point, NY 11050
(516) 944-8900   (516) 944-8637 (TTY)
FAX (516) 944-7302
www.helenkeller.org/national

Offers evaluation, vocational rehabilitation training, counseling, job preparation, placement, and related services through ten regional offices. Newsletter, "NAT-CENT News," published three times FREE to individuals who are deaf-blind and libraries; all others, $10.00.

LIGHTHOUSE INTERNATIONAL
111 East 59th Street
New York, NY 10022
(800) 334-5497 (V/TTY)   (212) 821-9200
(212) 821-9713 (TTY)   FAX (212) 821-9705
www.lighthouse.org

Provides information on vision problems faced by older people and how these problems can be treated. Makes referrals to local support groups throughout the U.S. for adults who are visually impaired or blind. Sells community education materials. Also available on the web site. Conducts conferences and training programs. Newsletter, "Aging and Vision News," published two times a year. FREE. Also available on the web site.

MACULAR DEGENERATION FOUNDATION (MDF)
PO Box 531313
Henderson, NV
(888) 633-3937   www.eyesight.org

Provides information and support for individuals with macular degeneration. Produces e-mail newsletter, "The Magnifier."

MACULAR DEGENERATION INTERNATIONAL
6700 North Oracle Road, #505
Tucson, AZ 85704
(800) 393-7634   (520) 797-2525
FAX (520) 797-8018   www.maculardegeneration.org

Support network for individuals with early or late onset macular degeneration. Membership, $25.00, includes semi-annual LARGE PRINT newsletter, a LARGE PRINT resource guide, and an audio-cassette with "Information and Inspiration."

MEDLINEPLUS: VISION DISORDERS AND BLINDNESS
www.nlm.nih.gov/medlineplus/visiondisordersblindness.html

This web site provides links to sites for general information about vision disorders and blindness, symptoms and diagnosis, treatment, specific aspects of the condition, clinical trials, statistics, organizations, directories, and research. Includes eye disease simulations and information for seniors. Some information is available in Spanish. Provides links to MEDLINE research articles and related MEDLINEplus pages.

NATIONAL ASSOCIATION FOR VISUALLY HANDICAPPED (NAVH)
22 West 21st Street
New York, NY 10010
(212) 889-3141   FAX (212) 727-2931
www.navh.org

Sells LARGE PRINT books and low vision aids. Produces three LARGE PRINT newsletters, "Seeing Clearly," "In Focus" (for youths), and "navh UPDATE;" FREE. Membership, $50.00, includes discounts on purchases and use of library books by mail; limited membership, $25.00 (no library privileges). FREE catalogue ($2.50 donation requested).

NATIONAL EYE INSTITUTE (NEI)
Building 31, Room 6A32
2020 Vision Place
Bethesda, MD 20892
(301) 496-5248   www.nei.nih.gov

This federal agency conducts basic and clinical research on the causes and cures of eye diseases. Distributes brochures on eye diseases and conditions, such as age-related macular degeneration, cataract, diabetic retinopathy, and glaucoma, FREE. NEI also recruits patients as subjects for a variety of clinical studies. Referrals from ophthalmologists are necessary for enrollment in an appropriate study.

NATIONAL FEDERATION OF THE BLIND (NFB)
1800 Johnson Street
Baltimore, MD 21230
(410) 659-9314   FAX (410) 685-5653
www.nfb.org

National membership organization with chapters in many states. Provides information about available services, laws, and evaluation of new technology. Holds state and national annual conventions. Sponsors "Newsline," an electronic, synthetic speech newspaper service, and "America's Jobline," an employment database, accessed by touchtone telephone. Regular membership starts at $10.00. Publishes the "Braille Monitor," a monthly magazine available in standard print and alternate formats.

$25.00 a year contribution requested. Also available on the web site.

NATIONAL LIBRARY SERVICE FOR THE BLIND AND PHYSICALLY HANDICAPPED (NLS)
1291 Taylor Street, NW
Washington, DC 20542
(800) 424-8567 or 8572 (Reference Section)
(202) 707-5100   (202) 707-0744 (TTY)
FAX (202) 707-0712   www.loc.gov/nls

National library service that serves individuals in the U.S. and U.S. residents living abroad. Regional libraries in many states. Individuals must be unable to read standard print due to visual impairment or physical disability. Provides publications on 4-track audiocassette and flexible disc and the machines to play them, FREE. "Facts: Books for Blind and Physically Handicapped Individuals" describes NLS programs and eligibility requirements. "Talking Book Topics," published bimonthly, in alternate formats and on the web site, lists titles recently added to the national collection which are available through the network of regional libraries. All services and publications from NLS are FREE. Each state has at least one NLS regional library; call for information. Some NLS libraries distribute LARGE PRINT books.

PREVENT BLINDNESS AMERICA
500 East Remington Road
Schaumburg, IL 60173
(800) 331-2020   (847) 843-2020
FAX (847) 843-8458   www.prevent-blindness.org

This organization sponsors vision screenings. Local and state affiliates. Publications related to diseases and eye injuries, including some in LARGE PRINT and Spanish. FREE catalogue.

Newsletter, "Prevent Blindness News," $12.00; FREE sample available on the web site.

RECORDING FOR THE BLIND AND DYSLEXIC (RFB&D)
20 Roszel Road
Princeton, NJ 08540
(800) 221-4792   (609) 452-0606
www.rfbd.org

Records educational materials on four-track audiocassette for people who are legally blind or have physical or perceptual disabilities. Requires certification of disability by a medical or educational professional. Registration fee, $75.00, plus $25.00 annual membership fee. Sells four-track audiocassette players. Catalogue of books is available on the web site. Newsletter, "RFB&D News" published twice a year. FREE

RESOURCES FOR REHABILITATION
22 Bonad Road
Winchester, MA 01890
(781) 368-9094   FAX (781) 368-9096
www.rfr.org

Provides custom designed training programs for professionals and the public. Publishes the "Living with Low Vision Series," described below, under "PUBLICATIONS AND TAPES."

VISION COMMUNITY SERVICES
23A Elm Street
Watertown, MA 02472
(617) 926-4232   In MA, (800) 852-3029
FAX (617) 926-1412   www.mablind.org

Information center for individuals with sight loss. Publishes materials in LARGE PRINT and audiocassette, including the

"VISION Community Services Resource List" and "VISION Community Services Resource Update," a bimonthly resource newsletter; both are FREE.

COPING WITH LOW VISION
by Marshall E. Flax, Don J. Golembiewski, and Bette L. McCaulley
Thomson Learning
PO Box 6904
Florence, KY 41022
(800) 347-7707   FAX (859) 647-5023
www.thomsonlearning.com

This book discusses low vision, vision rehabilitation services, low vision aids, and community resources. LARGE PRINT, $22.95. Also available on 4-track audiocassette from National Library Service for the Blind and Physically Handicapped regional libraries, RC 38113.

COPING WITH THE DIAGNOSIS OF SIGHT LOSS
Resources for Rehabilitation
22 Bonad Road
Winchester, MA 01890
(781) 368-9094   FAX (781) 368-9096
www.rfr.org

Three consumers discuss their reactions and experiences when told that they were losing their vision. Audiocassette, $12.00 plus $3.00.

DIALOGUE
Blindskills, Inc.
Box 5181
Salem, OR 97304
(800) 860-4224   (503) 581-4224
FAX (503) 581-1078   www.blindskills.com

Quarterly magazine with information on technology and other resources, interviews, poetry, recipes, and an announcements section. Published in alternate formats. Legally blind readers, $28.00; others, $40.00.

THE ENCOUNTER
Carmichael Audio-Video Duplication
1025 South Saddleback Creek Road
Omaha, NE 68106
(402) 556-5677   FAX (402) 556-5416

This videotape, produced by the Nebraska Department of Public Institutions, depicts interactions between people with normal vision and those who are blind. The tape uses humor to show how people who are blind are capable of independent activities; it also addresses education and employment opportunities. 11 minutes. $8.50

IF BLINDNESS STRIKES: DON'T STRIKE OUT
by Margaret Smith
Charles C. Thomas, Publisher
2600 South First Street
Springfield, IL 62794-9265
(800) 258-8980   (217) 789-8980
FAX (217) 789-9130   www.ccthomas.com

Written by a rehabilitation counselor who is visually impaired, this book describes many adaptations and strategies for living with vision loss. Hardcover, $54.95; softcover, $38.95. Also available on 4-track audiocassette on loan from the National Library Service for the Blind and Physically Handicapped regional libraries, RC 21060. To purchase standard ($18.00) or 4-track ($6.00) audiocassettes, contact Readings for the Blind, 29451 Greenfield Road, Suite 216, Southfield, MI 48076; (248) 557-7776.

LIVING WELL WITH MACULAR DEGENERATION
by Bruce P. Rosenthal and Kate Kelley
Penguin Putnam, Inc.
(800) 788-6262   www.penguinputnam.com

This book discusses the symptoms and causes of macular degeneration, describes vision rehabilitation, and provides information about simple and complex assistive devices. Includes chapter on driving and other options. $12.95

LIVING WITH LOW VISION SERIES
Resources for Rehabilitation
22 Bonad Road
Winchester, MA 01890
(781) 368-9094   FAX (781) 368-9096
www.rfr.org

A series of publications for individuals with vision loss and professionals who serve them. (See order form on last page of this book.)

LARGE PRINT publications for distribution by professionals to people with vision loss. Titles include "How to Keep Reading with Vision Loss," "Aids for Everyday Living with Vision Loss," and disease specific titles. See last page of this book for a complete list of titles and prices.

"Living with Low Vision: A Resource Guide for People with Sight Loss"
A comprehensive directory that helps people with sight loss locate services they need to remain independent. Describes products that enable people to keep reading, working, and carrying out their daily activities. LARGE PRINT. $46.95

"Meeting the Needs of People with Vision Loss: A Multidisciplinary Perspective"
by Susan L. Greenblatt (ed.)
Written by rehabilitation professionals, physicians, and a sociologist, this book discusses how to provide appropriate information and how to serve special populations, including people with diabetes and vision loss; elders with hearing loss and vision loss; and elders in long term care facilities. Includes a series of Multidisciplinary Case Studies. Also available on audiocassette. $24.95

"Providing Services for People with Vision Loss: A Multidisciplinary Perspective"
by Susan L. Greenblatt (ed.)
Written by ophthalmologists and rehabilitation professionals, this book discusses the need to provide coordinated care for people with vision loss. Also available on audiocassette. $19.95

MACULAR DEGENERATION SOURCE BOOK
by Bert Glaser and Lester A. Picker
Addicus Books, Inc.
PO Box 45327
Omaha, Ne 68145
(800) 352-2873   (402) 330-7493
FAX (402) 330-7493   www.AddicusBooks.com

This book describes the symptoms, diagnosis, and treatment of macular degeneration. It discusses the emotional impact; gives tips for coping; and describes accommodations in the home, workplace, and for travel and recreation. Includes resource list and glossary. $14.95

MAKING LIFE MORE LIVABLE
AFB Press
PO Box 1020
Sewickley, PA 15143
(800) 232-3044   FAX (412) 741-0609
www.afb.org

Offers simple adaptations to make the home safer for people with visual impairment. Available in LARGE PRINT and disk. $24.95

NATIONAL EYE INSTITUTE (NEI)
Building 31, Room 6A32
2020 Vision Place
Bethesda, MD 20892
(301) 496-5248   www.nei.nih.gov

NEI distributes booklets that discuss the causes, treatments, and research for major eye disorders such as cataract, diabetic retinopathy, glaucoma, and age-related macular degeneration. Some are available in LARGE PRINT from NEI (FREE) and on audiocassette ($2.00) from VISION Community Services, 23A Elm Street, Watertown, MA 02472. Also available on the web site.

THE NEW WHAT DO YOU DO WHEN YOU SEE A BLIND PERSON?
AFB Press
PO Box 1020
Sewickley, PA 15143
(800) 232-3044   FAX (412) 741-0609
www.afb.org

This videotape offers tips on interacting with individuals who are blind or visually impaired. 16 minutes. Also available with open captioning or audio description. $39.95

OUT OF THE CORNER OF MY EYE: LIVING WITH VISION LOSS IN
LATER LIFE
by Nicolette Pernod Ringgold
AFB Press
PO Box 1020
Sewickley, PA 15143
(800) 232-3044   FAX (412) 741-0609
www.afb.org

Written by a woman who became legally blind due to macular
degeneration in her late 70s, this book offers practical advice and
encouragement for elders with vision loss. LARGE PRINT and
audiocassette. $24.95

PROFILES IN AGING AND VISION
by Alberta L. Orr
AFB Press
PO Box 1020
Sewickley, PA 15143
(800) 232-3044   FAX (412) 741-0609
www.afb.org

This videotape provides information about the eye conditions
common in elders and services which promote independent
living. 33 minutes. $39.95

SEE FOR YOURSELF
Lighthouse International
111 East 59th Street
New York, NY 10022
(800) 334-5497 (V/TTY)   (212) 821-9200
(212) 821-9713 (TTY)   FAX (212) 821-9705
www.lighthouse.org

This videotape portrays elders with vision loss living independently using low vision aids and other assistive devices. Closed captioned. Available in English and Spanish. $50.00

SHARING SOLUTIONS
Lighthouse International
111 East 59th Street
New York, NY 10022
(800) 334-5497 (V/TTY)   (212) 821-9200
(212) 821-9713 (TTY)   FAX (212) 821-9705
www.lighthouse.org

Published twice a year, this newsletter makes suggestions for coping with limited vision and provides a forum for support group members to share information. FREE. Available in alternate formats and on the web site.

SOCIAL SECURITY: IF YOU ARE BLIND OR HAVE LOW VISION - HOW WE CAN HELP
Social Security Administration
(800) 772-1213   (800) 325-0778 (TTY)
www.ssa.gov

This publication provides information about obtaining Social Security benefits. The Social Security Administration distributes many other titles, including those that are available in standard print, alternate formats, and on the web site. Also available at local Social Security offices. (See Chapter 2, "PUBLICATIONS AND TAPES" section, for other titles available from the Social Security Administration.)

SOLUTIONS FOR EVERYDAY LIVING FOR OLDER PEOPLE WITH VISUAL IMPAIRMENTS
by Alberta L. Orr and Priscilla A. Rogers
Lighthouse International
111 East 59th Street
New York, NY 10022
(800) 334-5497 (V/TTY)   (212) 821-9200
(212) 821-9713 (TTY)   FAX (212) 821-9705
www.lighthouse

This videotape shows how staff can support independent living for residents in continuing care communities and other housing sites for elders. Describes various types of vision loss and illustrates adaptive strategies. 34 minutes. $59.95

TAKE CHARGE OF YOUR LIFE WITH VISION REHABILITATION
Lighthouse International
111 East 59th Street
New York, NY 10022
(888) 770-7660   FAX (800) 368-4111
www.lighthouse.org

This publication offers practical information for living independently with visual impairment. LARGE PRINT. $10.95

TALKING BOOKS FOR SENIOR ADULTS
National Library Service for the Blind and Physically Handicapped (NLS)
1291 Taylor Street NW
Washington, DC 20542
(800) 424-8567 (to receive application)
(202) 707-5100   (202) 707-0744 (TTY)
FAX (202) 707-0712   www.loc.gov/nls

This brochure promotes the use of talking books by seniors and describes how to receive them. Available in English and Spanish. FREE

THROUGH GRANDPA'S EYES
by Patricia MacLachlan
Harper Collins Publishers
PO Box 588
Scranton, PA 18512
(800) 331-3761   www.harpercollins.com

In this children's story, a young boy learns how his grandfather sees by using his senses of hearing, touch, and smell. $15.89. Also available on audiocassette on loan from the National Library Service for the Blind and Physically Handicapped regional libraries, RC 25436.

UNDERSTANDING AND LIVING WITH GLAUCOMA: A REFERENCE GUIDE FOR PATIENTS AND THEIR FAMILIES
Glaucoma Research Foundation
200 Pine Street, Suite 200
San Francisco, CA 94104
(800) 826-6693   (415) 986-3162
FAX (415) 986-3763   www.glaucoma.org

Written by a person with glaucoma, this booklet describes living with a chronic health condition. Single copy, FREE.

VISION SELF-HELP GROUP MEETING
Resources for Rehabilitation
22 Bonad Road
Winchester, MA 01890
(781) 368-9094   FAX (781) 368-9096
www.rfr.org

Audiocassette of a self-help group of individuals who are visually impaired discussing common problems and solutions for every-day living with vision loss. $12.00

THE WORLD THROUGH THEIR EYES
Lighthouse International
111 East 59th Street
New York, NY 10022
(800) 334-5497 (V/TTY)   (212) 821-9200
(212) 821-9713 (TTY)   FAX (212) 821-9705
www.lighthouse.org

This videotape portrays elders with vision loss living in a long term care facility and shows how staff can enhance residents' independence through the use of assistive devices such as low vision aids. Accompanying manual discusses common types of visual impairment. $25.00

RESOURCES FOR ASSISTIVE DEVICES

Listed below are publications that provide information about assistive devices and catalogues that specialize in devices for people with vision loss. Generic catalogues that sell some aids for people with vision loss are listed in Chapter 3, "MAKING EVERYDAY LIVING SAFER AND EASIER." Unless otherwise noted, the catalogues are FREE.

ANN MORRIS ENTERPRISES
551 Hosner Mountain Road
Stormville, NY 12582
(800) 454-3175   (845) 227-9659
FAX (845) 226-2793   www.annmorris.com

Catalogue available in alternate formats. Braille catalogue, $10.00. Also available on the web site.

FLORIDA NEW CONCEPTS MARKETING
PO Box 261
Port Richey, FL 34673
(800) 456-7097   FAX (727) 842-3231 (V/FAX)
gulfside.com/compulenz

Sells CompuLenz, which fits on most computer monitors, and enlarges character size while eliminating distortion and light reflection. Prices vary with monitor size.

INDEPENDENT LIVING AIDS, INC. (ILA)
200 Robbins Lane
Jericho, NY 11753
(800) 537-2118   FAX (516) 752-3135
www.independentliving.com

Catalogue is available in standard print, alternate formats, and on the web site.

LS & S GROUP
PO Box 673
Northbrook, IL 60065
(800) 468-4789   (800) 317-8533 (TTY)
FAX (847) 498-1482   www.lssgroup.com

Standard print catalogue.

MONS INTERNATIONAL
6595 Roswell, NE, #224
Atlanta, GA 30328
(800) 541-7903   www.magnifiers.com

LARGE PRINT catalogue.

NATIONAL FEDERATION OF THE BLIND
Materials Center
1800 Johnson Street
Baltimore, MD 21230
(410) 659-9314   FAX (410) 685-5653
www.nfb.org

Catalogue available in standard print, alternate formats, and on the web site.

VISUAL AIDS AND INFORMATIONAL MATERIAL
National Association for Visually Handicapped (NAVH)
22 West 21st Street
New York, NY 10010
(212) 889-3141   FAX (212) 727-2931
www.navh.org

LARGE PRINT catalogue; members, FREE; nonmembers, $2.50 donation requested. Also available on the web site.

INDEX OF ORGANIZATIONS

This index contains only those organizations listed under sections titled "ORGANIZATIONS." These organizations may also be listed as vendors of publications, tapes, and other products.

PUBLICATIONS FROM RESOURCES FOR REHABILITATION

Resources for Elders with Disabilities

This LARGE PRINT resource directory provides information about the services and products that elders with disabilities need to function independently. This book includes information on the diseases that cause common disabilities; the major rehabilitation networks; self-help groups; and legislation that affects people with disabilities. Chapters on hearing loss, vision loss, diabetes, arthritis, osteoporosis, Parkinson's disease, and stroke describe assistive devices, organizations, and publications. Plus information about aids for everyday living, falls, travel, and housing. Includes Internet resources.

Fifth edition   ISBN 0-929718-31-3 $51.95

A Woman's Guide to Coping with Disability

This **unique** book addresses the special needs of women with disabilities and chronic conditions, such as social relationships, sexual functioning, pregnancy, childrearing, caregiving, and employment. Special attention is paid to ways in which women can advocate for their rights with the health care and rehabilitation systems. Written for women in all age categories, the book has chapters on the disabilities that are most prevalent in women or likely to affect the roles and physical functions unique to women. Included are arthritis, diabetes, epilepsy, lupus, multiple sclerosis, osteoporosis, and spinal cord injury. Each chapter also includes information about the condition, service providers, and psychological aspects plus descriptions of organizations, publications and tapes, and special assistive devices.

Third edition 2000   ISBN 0-929718-26-7 $44.95

(CONTINUED ON NEXT PAGE)

A Man's Guide to Coping with Disability

Written to fill the void in the literature regarding the special needs of men with disabilities, this book includes information about men's responses to disability, with a special emphasis on the values men place on independence, occupational achievement, and physical activity. Information on finding local services, self-help groups, laws that affect men with disabilities, sports and recreation, and employment is applicable to men with any type of disability or chronic condition. The disabilities that are most prevalent in men or that affect men's special roles in society are included. Chapters on coronary heart disease, diabetes, HIV/AIDS, multiple sclerosis, prostate conditions, spinal cord injury, and stroke include information about the disease or condition, psychological aspects, sexual functioning, where to find services, environmental adaptations, and annotated entries of organizations, publications and tapes, and resources for assistive devices. Includes Internet resources.
Second edition 1999   ISBN 0-929718-23-2 $44.95

Making Wise Medical Decisions
How to Get the Information You Need

This book includes a **wealth** of information about where to go and what to read in order to make wise medical decisions. The book describes a plan for obtaining relevant health information and evaluating medical tests and procedures, health care providers, and health facilities. Each chapter includes extensive resources to help the reader get started. Chapters include Getting the Information You Need to Make Wise Medical Decisions; Locating Appropriate Health Care; Asking the Right Questions About Medical Tests and Procedures; Protecting Yourself in the Hospital; Medical Benefits and Legal Rights; Drugs; Protecting the Health of Children Who Are Ill; Special Issues Facing Elders; People with Chronic Illnesses and Disabilities and the Health Care System; Making Decisions About Current Medical Controversies; and Terminal Illness.
Second edition 2001   ISBN 0-929718-29-1 $42.95

Meeting the Needs of Employees with Disabilities

A comprehensive resource guide that provides information to help people with disabilities retain or obtain employment. Includes information on government programs and laws such as the Americans with Disabilities Act. Chapters on hearing and speech impairments, mobility impairments, visual impairment and blindness describe organizations, environmental adaptations, adaptive equipment, and services plus suggestions for a safe and friendly workplace. Case vignettes describing accommodations for employees with disabilities are an added feature of this special volume.

Third edition 1999   ISBN 0-929718-25-9 $44.95

Resources for People with Disabilities and Chronic Conditions

A comprehensive resource guide with chapters on spinal cord injury, low back pain, diabetes, multiple sclerosis, hearing and speech impairments, vision impairment and blindness, and epilepsy. Each chapter includes information about the disease or condition; psychological aspects of the condition; professional service providers; environmental adaptations; assistive devices; and descriptions of organizations, publications, and products. Chapters on rehabilitation services, independent living, self-help, laws that affect people with disabilities (including the ADA), and making everyday living easier. Special information for children is also included.

Fifth edition 2002   ISBN 0-929718-30-5 $56.95

Living with Low Vision:
A Resource Guide for People with Sight Loss

The only LARGE PRINT comprehensive guide to services and products that help individuals with vision loss. An extremely valuable self-help tool, this guide provides people with sight loss the information they need to keep reading, working, and enjoying life. Chapters on self-help groups, making everyday living easier, and special information for children, elders, and people with vision loss and hearing loss. Information on laws that affect people with vision loss, including the ADA, and high tech equipment that promotes independence and employment. Includes Internet resources.

Sixth edition 2001   ISBN 0-929718-28-3 $46.95

Providing Services for People with Vision Loss
A Multidisciplinary Perspective
Susan L. Greenblatt, Editor

Written by ophthalmologists, rehabilitation professionals, a physician who has experienced vision loss, and a sociologist, this book discusses how various professionals can work together to provide coordinated care for people with vision loss. Chapters include Vision Loss: A Patient's Perspective; Vision Loss: An Ophthalmologist's Perspective; Operating a Low Vision Aids Service; The Need for Coordinated Care; Making Referrals for Rehabilitation Services; Mental Health Services: The Missing Link; Self-Help Groups for People with Sight Loss; Aids and Techniques that Help People with Vision Loss; plus a Glossary. Also available on audiocassette.

1989   ISBN 0-929718-02-X $19.95

Meeting the Needs of People with Vision Loss
A Multidisciplinary Perspective
Susan L. Greenblatt, Editor

Written by rehabilitation professionals, physicians, and a sociologist, this book discusses how to provide appropriate information and how to serve special populations. Chapters include What People with Vision Loss Need to Know; Information and Referral Services for People with Vision Loss; The Role of the Family in the Adjustment to Blindness or Visual Impairment; Diabetes and Vision Loss - Special Considerations; Special Needs of Children and Adolescents; Older Adults with Vision and Hearing Losses; Providing Services to Visually Impaired Elders in Long Term Care Facilities; plus a series of Multidisciplinary Case Studies. Also available on audiocassette.

1991   ISBN 0-929718-07-0 $24.95

LARGE PRINT PUBLICATIONS

Designed for distribution by professionals, these publications include information on the specific disability or chronic condition, rehabilitation services, service providers, products, and resources that help people to live independently. Titles include "Living with Low Vision," "Living with Diabetes", "How to Keep Reading with Vision Loss," and "Living with Age-Related Macular Degeneration. Printed in 18 point bold type on ivory paper with black ink for maximum contrast. 8 1/2" by 11" Sold in minimum quantities of 25 copies per title. See order form on last page of this book for complete list of titles and prices.

See next page for order form

RESOURCES for REHABILITATION →

22 Bonad Road, Winchester, MA 01890
(781) 368-9094 FAX (781) 368-9096 e-mail: orders@rfr.org www.rfr.org
Our Federal Employer Identification Number is 04-2975-007

NAME _____

ORGANIZATION _____

ADDRESS _____

PHONE _____

[ ] Check or signed institutional purchase order enclosed for full amount of order. Purchase orders accepted from government agencies, hospitals, and universities <u>only</u>.

[ ] Mastercard/VISA Card number: _____

Signature: _____ Expiration date: _____

ALL ORDERS OF $50.00 OR LESS <u>MUST</u> BE PREPAID.

TITLE	QUANTITY	PRICE	TOTAL
Resources for elders with disabilities	____ X	$51.95	_____
Living with low vision: A resource guide	____ X	46.95	_____
Resources for people with disabilities and chronic conditions	____ X	56.95	_____
Meeting the needs of employees with disabilities	____ X	44.95	_____
A woman's guide to coping with disability	____ X	44.95	_____
A man's guide to coping with disability	____ X	44.95	_____
Making wise medical decisions	____ X	42.95	_____
The mental health resource guide	____ X	39.95	_____
Providing services for people with vision loss	____ X	19.95	_____
[ ] Check here for audiocassette edition			
Meeting the needs of people with vision loss	____ X	24.95	_____
[ ] Check here for audiocassette edition			

<u>MINIMUM PURCHASE OF 25 COPIES PER TITLE FOR THE FOLLOWING PUBLICATIONS</u>
Call for discount on purchases of 100 or more copies of any single title.

Living with low vision	____ X	2.00	_____
How to keep reading with vision loss	____ X	1.75	_____
Living with diabetic retinopathy	____ X	1.75	_____
Living with age-related macular degeneration	____ X	1.25	_____
Aids for everyday living with vision loss	____ X	1.25	_____
High tech aids for people with vision loss	____ X	1.75	_____
Living with diabetes	____ X	1.75	_____
		SUB-TOTAL	_____

SHIPPING & HANDLING: $50.00 or less, add $5.00; $50.01 to 100.00, add $8.00; add $4.00 for each additional $100.00 or fraction of $100.00. Alaska, Hawaii, U.S. territories, and Canada, add $3.00 to shipping and handling charges. Foreign orders must be prepaid in U.S. currency. Please write for shipping charges.

S/H	_____
TOTAL	$ _____

<u>Prices are subject to change.</u>